A Young Man's Journey with AIDS

The Story of Nick Trevor

A Young Man's Journey with AIDS

The Story of Nick Trevor

by

Luellen K. Reese

Franklin Watts

New York • London • Hong Kong • Sydney
Danbury, Connecticut

Photographs © Luellen Reese

Library of Congress Cataloging-in-Publication Data
Reese, Luellen K.
A young man's journey with AIDS: the story of Nick Trevor /
by Luellen K. Reese.
p.   cm.   —(Lesbian and gay expereince)
Includes bibliographical references and index.
Summary: The mother of a young man with AIDS tells his story based on
the journal which she kept through their experiences with his illness.
ISBN 0-531-11366-3
1. Trevor, Nicholas J. —Health.   2. AIDS (Disease) in adolescence —
Patients — United States — Biography. [1. Trevor, Nicholas, J. 2. AIDS
(Disease) 3. Diseases.]   I. Title.   II. Series
RJ387.A25R44   1997
362.1'969792'0092 — dc21
[B]
                                                              97-21622
                                                                   CIP
                                                                    AC

Printed in the United States of America. Published simultaneously in Canada
1 2 3 4 5 6 7 8 9 10 R 06 05 04 03 02 01 00 99 98 97

Contents

A Young Man's Journey with AIDS

The Story of Nick Trevor

Foreword

Several years ago a friend bemoaned the latest AIDS headline. "This is horrible," he said. "Fifty thousand people in this country have died of AIDS."

"That's a tragedy," I replied, "but let's put it into perspective. After all, 50,000 women in this country die of breast cancer each year."

"Yes." My friend nodded. "But that number is going to get smaller."

One hundred thousand deaths later, my own son was diagnosed with AIDS. Since then, another 300,000 people in this country have died of this disease. For a while, it seemed as though the number of new HIV infections might level off, or even decrease, but unfortunately this has not been the case. The number of young people between the ages of fifteen and nineteen who are being infected continues to grow. AIDS kills one in three black men between the ages of twenty-seven and forty-nine, and one in five black women in that same age group. As much as we try to ignore it, it doesn't go away.

Seventeen years into this epidemic there remains an

abundance of ignorance about the disease. People are still confused as to how it is contracted, what it does, how to behave around someone who has it. There is, I found as I accompanied my son on his journey with AIDS, a terrible, putrid stigma attached to this disease that hobbles our best personal and public efforts to deal with it. This stigma makes it hard for people—parents and children, teachers and students—to talk about it. In 1993, the number of teenagers infected by this disease increased 53 percent! We need to talk about it. To quote the Act Up slogan, "Silence equals death."

When my son was well enough, he often spoke to groups of young people about AIDS. The young people who heard him speak were always moved by his story because he was one of them. He was a teenager when he was infected. Seeing him, a person with AIDS, stand before them made the disease real. Seeing him made it seem possible that they might be at risk if they were not cautious. He was sometimes able to dispel some of the uninformed prejudices they had about people with AIDS, people who are, after all, just people.

In his memory, I have chosen to share his story with young people so that they may learn from his experiences. It is my hope that after having read this story, its readers will know more about AIDS, how it is contracted, what the disease is like, and what it is like to have a disease that has no cure and is accompanied by a stigma, even today.

I have written the story in the third person from my son's point of view, which was possible to do because he had been so honest with me and because I had kept a journal throughout our experience with his illness. I wrote this story in honor of my son, all those who have died of AIDS, and those millions who still fight.

Throughout it all, *I have wanted to write it all down, to give it a name, to be able to let fingers run through it. Perhaps I can make it more tangible, substantive, real to me, and to anyone who cares to know. This is my story. It has a beginning, because there's never any end.*

Nicolas J. Trevor
1993

Young people have always taken on an air of immortality, of invincibility. When the transmission path for Acquired Immunodeficiency Syndrome (AIDS) became known, adults, by and large, changed their behaviors. Youths, however, either didn't get the message or refused to listen to it. Patricia Fleming, director of the White House AIDS Policy Office, issued a call for action in the spring of 1996 with this warning: "Too many young people are putting themselves at risk. . . . And far too many are paying the ultimate price—premature death. Today in the United States, nearly half of all new infections are occurring among people under the age of 25 and nearly one-quarter of those new infections are among teenagers." (Keith Clark, "Federal Report on Youth and AIDS Shows Little Progress," *Gay and Lesbian Times*, March 7, 1996, p. 25) Nick Trevor was one who thought himself to be invincible.

CHAPTER ONE

It Can't Happen to Me

Nick Trevor had heard the facts. He knew all about AIDS. He knew what the dangers were, and yet, somehow he felt immune to all threats. *It can't happen to me,* he thought. *Grown-ups say that unsafe sex is dangerous. Grown-ups say doing drugs and sharing needles are foolhardy. What do they know? They're just trying to scare me out of having a good time.*

Nick had a good time. He lived life the way he wanted to. He made all the mistakes he felt entitled to make and never thought he would have to face up to their consequences. It is a cold truth that teaches life's mistakes are not so easily forgotten. And Nick had just been slapped in the face with that truth.

He eyed the telephone nervously as he contemplated the call he was about to make. Picking up the receiver he dialed his mother's work number.

"Mom, it's Nick," he said, trying to sound as normal as he could.

"Hi, sweetheart, what's going on?"

"I have some bad news." He was tentative. He had to tell

his mother, he wanted to tell his mother, but the words wouldn't flow.

"Okay, what is it?" she asked.

"I'm in the hospital," he said finally.

"What's wrong?"

Nick sensed his mother was tense. It was more than the tone of her voice, it was twenty-one years of being her son. "I have pneumonia," he said, pausing.

He didn't want to upset her. He found it difficult to deal with his mother when she was upset. He wanted her to receive calmly what he had to tell her, but he knew that was unlikely. "And the news might be worse than that," he continued.

There was a moment's silence on the phone before his mother spoke. "Tell me the whole thing," she said.

"Can you come and see me? I think I should tell you in person."

"Nick," his mother said impatiently, "tell me everything. I can't drive all the way up to the hospital not knowing."

"The kind of pneumonia I have is called *pneumocystic pneumonia*. Only people with cancer or AIDS get it." He stopped to take a breath and tried to imagine his mother's reaction. "They gave me an HIV test. The results aren't back yet, but we're one hundred percent sure it's what I've got."

"Let's not get excited until we know for sure," said his mother. "Maybe it's a mistake."

"Mom, it's not a mistake!" he said. Again he stopped to take a deep, labored breath. "Can you come visit me?"

Only a few days before, Nick and his girlfriend, Kim, had not a care in the world. They had been on a ride up the coast, headed for Oregon to visit Kim's best friend. Nick hadn't been feeling well for about three or four weeks, and along the way he had a coughing fit.

"Are you okay?" Kim asked. "Do you want me to drive?"

"No, I'm fine," he said, "I can drive." He didn't want Kim to worry. And he didn't want to be sick.

"You really should see a doctor," she said.

"I know. I called the clinic to make an appointment, but they can't see me for three more weeks."

They got as far as Eureka when Nick began to have trouble breathing. He just couldn't seem to fill his lungs up with air, and he was coughing.

"Nick, what is wrong?" Kim asked.

"It's getting hard to breathe," he said. He hesitated before saying what was on his mind. "I hope I don't have AIDS." There, I said it, he thought. Having said it, maybe it would go away.

"Nick, don't be silly. You couldn't have AIDS," Kim said. "Don't even say such a terrible thing."

Nick didn't say anything more. He knew Kim thought he was being dramatic, but he feared that what he had suspected for several weeks now was true.

"We better go home," said Kim.

Nick turned the car around and they headed south, stopping along the way to buy antihistamines, cough drops, and broncho inhalers, anything that might make it easier for Nick to breathe and stop coughing.

Several hours later they were back in San Jose. The next day they went straight to the county hospital where they sat in a crowded lobby for three hours waiting to see a health care professional. Kim had some errands to run, so she left Nick and went out for a while. When she got back, Nick was in an emergency room cubicle being admitted to the hospital. He had just been told he had AIDS.

When Kim came into the room, Nick knew the look on his face told her it was serious. "I have what I thought I had," he said, trying to sound as upbeat as possible.

✦

As Nick waited for his parents to get to the hospital, nurses and attendants settled him into his room and hooked him up to oxygen and an intravenous (IV) tube carrying a saline solution with medication into his bloodstream. Kim, at his bedside, looked very drained and scared. Nick was tired, but he felt relieved when his parents finally got there. Bill, Nick's dad, couldn't stay long, but Luellen, his mom, stayed for hours. Doctors and nurses came and went, all looking very somber. Finally, when Nick was a little more comfortable, Luellen went home. Kim stayed and slept on the floor by his bed.

The next day, at ten-thirty, Nick called his mother again. "Mom, can you come and see me right away?"

"I'm at work now," she said. "I was planning to come right after."

"The doctor was just here," he said breathlessly. The pneumonia filled his lungs with fluid, making it difficult for him to catch his breath. Almost gasping for air, he sounded as though he had just finished running a mile. "The news isn't good. If you wait until after work, I might not be here."

"What are you saying?" his mother asked cautiously.

"They said I'm much worse. I might not make it till tonight."

A short time later, Luellen walked into his room. She had driven the thirty-five miles to the hospital in thirty-five minutes. Nick was in reverse isolation. This meant all visitors to his room had to wear gowns, gloves, and masks. Nick had to be protected from all bacteria that might make him sicker. No one could touch Nick for fear of infecting him with some otherwise harmless germ that, in his weakened condition, could kill him. His white-cell count had fallen to below 300 (normal is 3600 and higher), and he was in serious danger of infection. He saw the look of terror on her face as his mother surveyed the room. "Calm down," he told her. "It will be all right."

His friend Dave came to see him. "Daveman" and "Nickman," as they called each other, chatted and joked as they had always done. Chatting with the Daveman was enjoyable, and for a while it all seemed almost regular to Nick, except that Dave and Luellen were wearing weird hospital garb and he had tubes going in and out of his nose and arms.

The third or fourth day Nicolas was in the hospital, the reality of what was happening to him set in, and he began to feel guilt. All his life, Nick had never made the connection between cause and effect, had never behaved as though what he did today would affect tomorrow. Now, his yesterdays were stealing his tomorrows. He was suddenly afraid and asked to see the Catholic chaplain.

"Father" was not what Nick expected, or needed. Retired from active parish work, Father volunteered at the hospital three days a week. Nick was touched by the compassion he could see the priest had for people with AIDS, but he was dismayed that Father saw it as his duty to encourage them to be sorry for their sins before they died. Father gave Nick the Anointing of the Sick, a sacrament of forgiveness and spiritual healing commonly given to those who are ill. Then he proceeded to tell Nick that it was a sin to be gay. By the time his mom arrived to visit him that evening, Nick was in a tempestuous mood.

"Mom, you'll be happy to hear that I saw a priest today," he said. Nick's voice was spiced with sarcasm.

"And what happened?"

"It was a big mistake. He gave me Last Rites, and then he told me it's a sin to be gay. We got into a big argument. He wanted me to confess things I don't think are sins. He wouldn't leave until I did, so I finally said whatever he wanted to hear just to get rid of him." Nick was frustrated at the priest's behavior, but not surprised.

"Nick, I'm sure you misunderstood him. The Catholic Church doesn't teach that it's a sin to *be* gay, only that certain things people who are gay might do are a sin."

"No, Mom, this priest said it's a sin to be gay."

"Well, he's wrong," she said.

He didn't want to argue with his mother so he changed the

subject. "Anyway, I had the Last Rites and nothing happened."

"What did you think was going to happen?" Luellen leaned against the side of the bed and stroked Nick's head.

"I don't know. I thought I would see God, or have a miraculous conversion or something." He smiled at his mother. He had lost his enthusiasm for the seriousness of the conversation and wanted to end it on a lighter note. He had told her he tried it her way, by talking to a priest, and now he hoped she would forget the whole incident.

On Saturday morning, the phone rang. It was Nick's mother. "Your father, your sister and grandfather, and I are coming to see you, today," she said.

When the family got to the hospital, Nick was feeling better. He was no longer in reverse isolation and his spirits were good. Bill and Luellen left the room for a few minutes so that Elizabeth and Nick could talk. Elizabeth was Nick's younger sister. They were as different as night and day, and he had never taken her seriously. Nick knew she lived in his shadow, had to deal with his traumas. It was only around the time of his twenty-first birthday, just a few months before, that they began to see each other as real people instead of irritating siblings.

Their grandfather started the conversation. "Maybe it's time the two of you put aside your differences and the ways of your childhood and started to relate to one another like adults," he said.

Nick lifted one hand slightly and let his fingers fall back into place across his chest. "Sure," he said.

Elizabeth started in earnest. "Nick," she said, "I know we've had a lot of fights and stuff, but I just want to say I'm sorry and I love you."

Nick could see that she was nervous. As she spoke, she

pulled at several strands of her long blond hair. Suddenly, he felt great compassion for his little sister. "I love you, too, Liz, and I'm sorry." He smiled at her.

Nick surprised his doctors. He didn't die, as they had expected, but started to get better and finally the doctors let him go home.

He arrived at his parents' house weighing 135 pounds, 30 pounds less than he should have weighed. But his white cell count was up to 1500, and he was improving. Every day, the visiting nurses came to administer an intravenous infusion of pentamadin, the medication used to treat *pneumocystic pneumonia* (PCP). He had a heplock in his arm, which the nurses used to insert the IV for the infusion.

As he began to recover from the pneumonia, Nick became interested in what his prognosis was. At first, his parents tried to hide it from him. Later he learned that the doctors had told them he had six, maybe nine, months at the most.

When Nick finally pried this information out of his mother, he was shaken. But Luellen told him, "Doctors don't know. How can they say for sure when a person is going to die? Don't pay any attention to how long they say you have to live." Yet, how could Nick not pay attention? He'd just been given a death sentence. He was twenty-one, and he had only six months left to live.

Nick and his family fell into a routine fairly quickly. In the morning, he flushed his heplock with a saline solution and his mother fixed his breakfast before going to work. She would come home at eleven-thirty to feed him milkshakes to get his blood sugar level up because the pentamadin made it drop. At twelve-thirty the nurses would take over and start the medication. While he was on the infusion, Nick would eat candy bars, also to keep his blood sugar level up. Every thirty minutes, the nurses checked his sugar level. He would finish his infusion around two-thirty. When Luellen got home from work at four, she would try to get him to eat a snack. Later, Kim would arrive and girlfriend and mother would try to get Nick to eat dinner. Sometimes he'd eat well; sometimes not. Before bed, he took a pile of vitamins, flushed his heplock again, and checked his blood sugar one more time.

Nick loved his mother very much, but often she would drive him to distraction. Living in his parents' home, which he thought of as the "prison of love," was not easy for him. The first Sunday Nick was home, Luellen went to Mass, as she usually did, and came home with a priest in tow.

When Nick saw the young priest, he was infuriated at his mother for this presumptive invasion of his privacy, but he kept his cool. The priest seemed like a nice guy. He was a musician and he lived in Pacifica, where Nick and Kim were planning to move as soon as he was well enough. The two talked for a while. The priest read a few passages from the Bible and gave Nick Communion. Then Luellen gave the good father a ride home.

As soon as they left, Nick's emotions came to a head. He seethed with anger because his mother had forced this priest on him. When his father suggested that Nick finish his orange juice, Nick exploded into a rage and threw the orange juice through the window, smashing it. Then he retreated to his room, where he began packing his clothes and demanding that Kim take him away. He declared that he would never have anything to do with his meddling parents again.

By the time his mother returned, Nick was completely exhausted, sitting on his bed amid a pile of clothes he had been trying to pack. Kim was sitting next to him, trying to soothe him.

"Nick, what are you doing?" Luellen asked.

"This isn't working," he railed. "You have no idea who I am. How could you do that to me?"

"Nick, I'm sorry," she said. "I had no right to bring the priest here without asking you first."

"I need to be who I am and you're always trying to make me be what you want. It's always been that way, Mom." He tried to get up, but he was too weak.

"Nick, I'm sorry. I thought Father could explain to you that the other priest was wrong. I was only trying to help. Please calm down."

"Nick, listen to your mom," interjected Kim. "Try to calm down."

Nick looked at Kim and then settled down a bit. Luellen continued, "Look, everyone is upset right now. Why don't you and Kim go for a ride, take the day off, and when you come back, things will be better. And I promise that I will never bring surprise guests home again, okay?"

When they returned that evening, it was as if nothing had happened.

Adolescence has never been an easy time. Today, many young people come from two-wage-earner families. They have rapid access to global problems and witness, almost first-hand, the camera's detachment as it looks at everything from murder on Miami streets to ethnic cleansing in Bosnia. Many schools have been stripped of budgets that might provide courses and counseling that could help them put a realistic and personal face on the negative images they're bombarded with on television, while others are hampered by conservative watchdog groups who inhibit them from doing their job of providing factual, straight-forward, unbiased information. It's no wonder that many young people get lost, rebelling against their parents and getting caught up in a world of drugs and sex.

Unfortunately, rebellion in today's world and trying to find one's self can lead to death. In a 1995 news release, the Centers for Disease Control reported more than 18,500 cases of AIDS to date in 13–24 year olds. (Karen Ocamb, "Gay and Lesbian Youth Emerge from Generational Shadows," *Gay & Lesbian Times*; August 10, 1995, p. 43).

CHAPTER TWO

Being Free

It seemed to Nick that his parents were always trying to make him be someone he wasn't. Nicolas, or Jonathan,
as he had been named at birth, was most often at odds with
his parents. He was bright, talented, sensitive, and his parents
told him so, often. This praise was not pleasing to him.
Jonathan Francis Reese didn't want praise. He wanted to be
his own person.

The desire to be his own person turned to expression
when, at fourteen, he announced he was changing his name
to "Nick Trevor." The name change wasn't a phase he would
outgrow, as he knew his parents thought. Nick Trevor was the
name of his freedom, and he was resolved to make it perma-
nent. In his sophomore year, he registered at a new school
using the name Nicolas Jonathan Trevor.

"Why are you doing this?" Luellen asked him. "Don't you
understand that your father and grandfather are very hurt that
you have rejected their name?"

"That's the point," Nick said quite matter-of-factly. "Reese
is their name. I want my own name. I'm not rejecting them.

I'm being me. I don't want to live in Dad's shadow and just be somebody's kid."

"Okay, be Nicolas Trevor," Luellen said, giving up.

"You can call me Jonathan, Mom. I'll still answer."

Being a musician was who Nick Trevor was. Music permeated every inch of his life. He listened to music, he played music, he wrote music. In the seventh grade, he won a full scholarship to the Bach Lyceum, a summer program for gifted young musicians. At his eighth grade graduation, he was honored as the most outstanding instrumental musician in the school, and he played an original composition on electric piano at the commencement.

In high school, he played snare drum in the marching band. Saturday mornings his mother drove him to practice and dropped him off at the front gate where the other kids were standing. As was his routine, he got out of the car, walked off, and stood ten to twelve feet away from the other band members.

One day, Luellen asked him, "Don't you have any friends in the band?"

"No," he answered. "They're all hayseeds." It was clear his mom didn't understand. It was written on her face. He didn't want to hang around with a bunch of guys who all looked the same.

Playing in the school band became less important to him when he met Alex. The two of them became fast friends and spent every spare moment at Alex's house writing and playing their own music. Nick relished the freedom of being master of his own music.

In his sophomore year, Nick ran away from home for the first time. His girlfriend, Samantha, moved to Pismo Beach with her family. Nicolas never just liked a girl. He always fell dramatically in love. He was, therefore, quite devastated when she left. He moped around for two weeks until she came to visit him for the weekend. When she arrived, he told his mother the two of them were going to sleep together.

"You cannot sleep with Samantha," Luellen said.

"Why not?" he demanded.

"Because you are only fifteen and she is only fourteen. You are too young to be sleeping together."

"*Her* parents don't care. They're cool. They'd let us sleep together. They'd trust us."

To Nick, it was a matter of trust and not of his parents' responsibility for his 14-year-old visitor. And he was dissatisfied when his mother's position did not change. So he and Samantha ran away to her house. There, they would be able to sleep together.

Nick was surprised that his parents let him stay there. He supposed they thought he'd get bored and come home on his own. Nick was right about Samantha's parents. They were very cool. They were so cool they not only let Nick and Samantha sleep together, but they didn't insist that Nick and Sam go to school and shared their marijuana with them. There was no way that Nick was going to get bored with this arrangement.

One day, though, they were sitting in Samantha's bedroom when they heard a knock at the front door. When Nick saw it was his dad, he ran out the back. The police, whom Bill had called to escort him to Samantha's house, grabbed Nick and held him. Bill removed the inside door handle from the passenger's side of his TR7, and the police helped deposit Nick into the seat. They immediately started the three hundred mile trip home.

His newly found independence suddenly snatched away from him, Nick was angry. He screamed at his father, threatened him and, once, tried to grab the steering wheel to swerve the car off the road. Bill said nothing.

It was the middle of the night when they reached their hometown. Nick knew his anger had frightened Bill, and he thought his anger had given him control of the situation. It hadn't. Bill didn't go home, but went to the local police station, instead.

The police took Nick into custody and put him in a foster home for the weekend. Although Bill and Luellen were to pick him up on Monday, Nick was so furious at his parents that he planned not to go home. The foster placement was just fine with him.

However on Monday, the police wouldn't let Nick go home. The police called a therapist the family had been seeing and it was decided that everyone should meet with him on Tuesday before a decision about the future would be made.

Nick was told that Bill and Luellen didn't know where he was. And he didn't know if they knew what kind of supervision or treatment he was being given. He had no way of contacting his parents and was allowed to think they had deliberately placed him in foster care and didn't want him home.

By Tuesday, Nick was not only angry, he was also very hurt. The session with the therapist did not go well and when the therapist asked Nick if he wanted to come home, he said, "No." It was exhilarating to be in control of whether or not he went home. It was a kind of freedom to him, to be able to choose between his home and a foster home, so he savored it.

The family met with the therapist the next Tuesday and the Tuesday after that, and each time the therapist had some new reason why Nick shouldn't go home. But Nick could see his mother was desperate. She wrung her hands, and her face was twisted with angst each week as she begged the therapist to let her son come home. Nick began to believe his parents wanted him, and he was becoming tired of his pseudo-freedom.

One Tuesday after the therapy session, the therapist let Luellen take Nick back to the foster home. "This is it," Nick said, as they pulled up to a ranch style house on a country road. "I hate it here. I want to get out."

"Dad and I are doing everything we can to get you out," said Luellen. "At least I know where you are now. If all else fails, maybe Dad and I can kidnap you."

"Just take me home now," Nick pleaded.

"I can't," Luellen explained. "They might take you away from us forever." She leaned across the seat and held him tight.

"Just do whatever you can," Nick said, as he got out of the car and walked into the group home. It was dawning on him that the cost of trying to be his own person was the loss of his independence. The fight for his freedom led him to be all but incarcerated with a band of cast-offs, juvenile criminals, and drug abusers.

The rules in the group home were strict, much stricter than the rules Nick faced at home. No one talked at the dinner table, and no one outwardly defied the authority of the couple running the home. Nick didn't trust either one of them. He tried to bide his time and waited for his release.

He shared a room with three other boys. One night after lights out, a twelve-year-old slipped out of his bunk and got into bed with an older kid. The two began to have sex with each other. Nick held his breath, pretending to be asleep, but he quietly watched. He was stunned and fascinated at the same time. He thought he should be repulsed, but he wasn't. He was curious and amazed.

A few nights later, two other boys came home from school with a pile of pills and a bottle of gin. It didn't take much encouragement for Nick to join them in the drinking and pill popping. As the affects of the dope and the booze began to set in, Nick started to feel free, free from the pain of his situation, free from the rules of the grown-up world — free. He relaxed. This is cool, he thought. He and the other boys started laughing and soon got carried away. They were making an awful racket and woke their custodians. The man of the house came in, discovered what the boys were up to, and called the police.

While the man and his wife turned on the lights, Nick started throwing up. He couldn't quite pay attention to what was going on. All he knew was that everyone was making a lot of noise. The police came and took the boys with the drugs away. A county social worker named Doug picked up Nick and took him home to his parents.

"There's been a big mistake," Nick heard Doug say to his father. His mother caught Nick as he stumbled and fell through the front door. "Your son should never have been in a group home."

Nick's mother took him into the bathroom and held his head while he vomited into the toilet. Then she took him into his room, put him on his bed, pulled off his shoes, and wiped his face with a damp wash cloth. "I love you, Jonathan," she said.

"I love you, too," Nick said. Then he passed out.

The time in the foster home changed Nick profoundly. After he got home, he felt different, almost numb. The cost of seeking to grab his freedom and be his own person without taking responsibility for that person was great. He lost whatever fear for his safety he may have had, and he learned to suppress his feelings so effectively it was several years before he could express any emotion except rage. It was no wonder, then, that he began cutting school and running away from home more frequently. He no longer cared what the consequences of his actions might be because he had endured the worst and survived it. He lost respect for his person, the person he wanted so desperately to be, and he began to live only for the thrill of the moment.

A couple of months later, during Christmas vacation, Nick was invited to an over-night party at the house of some of Alex's friends. There would be mostly people in their late teens and early twenties at the party, and Nick thought it was really cool to hang out with older kids. To prove he was one of them, he was determined to do whatever they did. There were a lot of drugs and alcohol at the party and Nicolas became so drunk, he blacked out. The next morning, he found himself in bed with Laura, a twen-

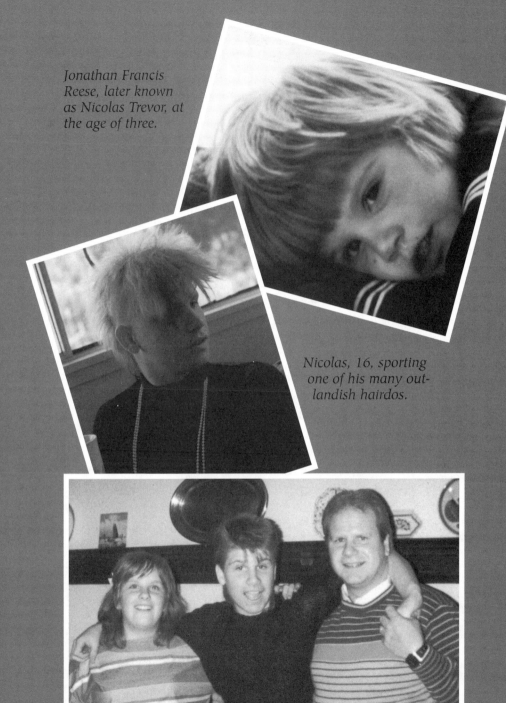

Jonathan Francis
Reese, later known
as Nicolas Trevor, at
the age of three.

Nicolas, 16, sporting
one of his many out-
landish hairdos.

Nicolas, 15, and his sister Elizabeth and his dad.

ty-four year old woman and Todd, a nineteen year old. Nick thought these adventures marked his independence and gave him control over his life. The thrill of having discovered sex added to his excitement.

After that, Nick began to dress weirdly, to wear makeup, and to fix his hair in the most outlandish ways. He began to push the limits of existence with reckless and contrary behavior, all as a demonstration of his freedom. There was nothing he would not try, just for the experience. This, he thought, was free self-expression.

A year or so later, he had a run-in with the police because he was truant. They asked him his name and he said, "Nicolas Trevor." The police took him to the station and called Bill to pick him up. When the police told Nick he had two choices, either go with his father or to juvenile hall, he again exercised his freedom of choice and refused to go home. Nick knew he would get in trouble for cutting school if he went home; he thought he would prefer to go to juvenile hall. The charge was lying to the police about his name.

The next day, he was released into the custody of his parents and given thirty days probation. Before his probation was up, he cut school again and was sent to juvenile hall.

Nick didn't usually like authority figures, especially ones connected with the justice system, but he liked his probation officer. He was cool and he agreed with Nick that Nick was not a criminal and did not belong in juvenile hall. The probation officer arranged for Nick to serve his time in a psychiatric hospital with a special program for troubled youth.

While in the hospital, Nick was subjected to all manner of physical and psychological testing, more encroachment upon his freedom. Because of his foray into the world of sex and drugs, Nick was given a test for HIV. The test was negative, but that did not mean he had not been infected. It meant that at that time, he didn't have HIV antibodies sufficient to show up in the test. He should have been tested again in six months. Considering the lifestyle he then espoused, he should have been tested every six months from that point on, but he wasn't.

It was then that his mother began to preach to him about the danger of AIDS, but he thought it was just another tool for her to use in trying to keep him in line. What did she know? he thought. She was just a mother, and she would do anything to keep him from being free.

Of course, the irony was that within a year, Nick's quest for freedom had led him to be incarcerated in, first, a foster home, then in juvenile hall, and finally in a psychiatric facility.

Often it is easier to deny reality than to deal with it, to deny concerns than to track down information. This is very true where AIDS/HIV is a concern, especially when there is a lack of agencies that exist specifically for youths. Outside of schools — and schools often perpetuate myths and misinformation when it comes to educating about AIDS — there are few agencies where young people can comfortably turn for testing, counseling, and information about prevention. It is simply easier and less embarrassing for young people in most parts of the United States and Canada to deny that there might be a problem or that they may be at risk of infection.

Sadly, many adults condone and perpetuate such denial by refusing to acknowledge that their children may be sexually active. They maintain that speaking out about sex will give young people ideas. But what generation of young people has not thought about sex? Without question, abstinence is the most effective way to avoid HIV/AIDS infection, but to deny that some teens are sexually active is to rush headlong through life with blinders on. "[T]hree quarters of American students say they have been sexually active by the time they leave high school." (Keith Clark, "Federal Report on Youth and AIDS Shows Little Progress, *Gay & Lesbian Times*, March 7, 1996, p. 25.)

CHAPTER THREE

The Two-edged Sword

Denial is a destructive as well as a useful tool. It can help one get through painful and difficult situations by closing one's eyes to what is really happening, and it can clog up reality so effectively that the situation persists and worsens the more it is denied. Denial became an important part of how Nick coped with the chaos in his life.

During the next two years, Nick was in and out of juvenile hall and the psychiatric hospital. He cut school so much that his counselor suggested he take the high school proficiency test and go to college, which he did. He ran away from home often and was frequently gone for weeks at a time. When he was on the streets, he did whatever he could to survive, including hustling (prostitution). When he'd come home, he'd have a few good weeks; then he'd get restless or upset with his parents and take off again.

He had, by then, many friends and was very popular with the outcast kids. Girls, especially, were always after him. Six or seven of them were usually sitting on the front lawn, waiting for him after school. Once a girl called him to ask for a date and he hung up on her. "Nick," Luellen said, "that was very unkind. You could have said no nicely. Why do you treat girls like they are a dime a dozen?"

He pointed out the window at the crowd of girls on the lawn and said, "Because they are." It was easy for Nick to deny the feelings of others when he was in such denial about his own feelings.

There was also a pack of boys two or three years younger than Nick who followed him around and copied everything he did. They dressed like him. If he changed his hair, the next day, they would be sporting new copies of his latest hairdo. His sister Elizabeth called them the "Nick-wanna-bes" and the name stuck.

He had real friends, too, mostly guys who were in his band. Alex, Daveman, Nickman, Paul, the artist, and Dylan, the poet, were the core group.

Part of the fog of denial that surrounded Nick was his belief that his life would be better, more exciting, if he were someplace else. When he turned eighteen, he went to live in San Francisco with a friend named Bob. They shared a room in a shabby boarding house in the Tenderloin, a seedy neighborhood in the Golden Gate City. It was a god-awful, flee-bitten place, but it was heaven to Nick because he was someplace else. He didn't stay there long, though. For about a year he floated back and forth between his parents' home and the floors of his friends' apartments. Finally, he settled in Haight-Ashbury with a beautiful, twenty year old girl named Melanie.

Melanie had been a model in New York for a few months when she was beaten by a man who mistook her for a prostitute. She told Nick the experience so scarred her that she ran all the way to San Francisco. Nick was attracted to her because of her vulnerability, the result of a heroin abusing mother and a father whom she never knew. Nick could see she didn't trust anyone, least of all men, and he was determined to change that. He tried to convince her that he was her soulmate, someone who understood her and listened to her, someone who cherished her. Nick was sure Melanie was "the one."

"What do you think of her?" he asked Luellen when she went to their flat to visit.

"She's very beautiful," Luellen said, "and very nice. I like her a lot and I think that the two of you will hurt each other very much."

Nick was confused and somewhat disappointed by his mother's answer. "Why do you say that?" he asked her.

"You're both too fragile, too dependent, and too co-dependent."

"I think you're wrong, Mom. She's the one," he insisted. Nick couldn't see, wouldn't see, the problem. He thought if you take enough drugs, drink enough, party enough, then everything will be all right. And Nick and Melanie lived a fast-paced life, full of parties, clubs, drugs, and sex.

Luellen confronted him with his drug abuse. "Listen, Nick, I wasn't born yesterday. You're losing weight, you stay up all night, night after night, you talk a mile a minute. You're on drugs."

"You're wrong," he answered, laughing and trying to make light of the assertion.

"Don't you know that drugs dilute who you are?" Luellen asked. "They're bad for you physically, mentally, and spiritually. You'll ruin your life if you don't stop."

"Mom, I swear to you I'm not on drugs. You're overreacting."

"You're speeding right now," she said.

Nick wondered how she knew. He straightened up and tried to look clean.

"There's no point in discussing it with you," his mother said. "I will say this, I will not support you in your own self-destruction. I'm not going to send you any more money, or help you, until you get clean and sober. If you decide you want to get off of drugs and you want help, your dad and I will do anything within our power to help you, but until then nothing."

"Okay, okay," he said, just glad that she wasn't going to talk about it anymore.

A couple of weeks later, Nick was so strung out on methamphetamines that Alex locked him in a room and wouldn't let him out until he called his parents for help. His mother answered the phone. "Mom," he said. His voice was shaky. It was uncomfortable admitting he was wrong, but he knew he had no choice. His drug problem was out of hand. "I'm calling you like you told me to. I need help."

Bill and Luellen raced to San Francisco and picked Nick up at Alex's apartment. Then they went to Nick's apartment to pick up a few of his things. Nick was so weak he could barely walk, but he insisted on going into his room with his father. Luellen waited outside. Melanie came out a few minutes later.

Soon, Bill and Nick came out of the apartment. Bill was carrying Nick's suitcase in one arm, and Nick was hanging on to the other arm. His head was down; he couldn't even look at Melanie.

The next day, his parents took Nick to a drug and alcohol rehabilitation hospital. He spent thirty days there being angry at his parents, himself, and the world. While he was there, he was tested again for HIV by an independent clinic. When he returned for the results, he was told they were inconclusive and his blood sample was being given a more definitive test. He was told to check again the following week. This, he determined, was because he must be positive and the people at the clinic didn't want to tell him. He called Luellen and told her he was ninety-nine percent sure he was HIV positive and asked her to come see him after work.

Nick was in his room when his mother arrived. His uneaten dinner was still on the tray, and he was lying in his bed crying. He looked up and reached out to her. Luellen climbed into the bed with him, held him in her arms, and rocked him back and forth. "Everything will be all right," she said. Nick felt safe in her arms.

Slowly, Nick came out of his depression and decided to go

to one of the twelve-step meetings in the hospital that night after his mother left. During the next few days, everything in his world began to get jumbled up and he was afraid. He was supposed to check back with the clinic for his test results, but he couldn't. Each day, he told himself not to worry. Each day, he became more and more convinced that this HIV thing was just some silly mistake. It couldn't happen to the Nickman.

His mother nagged him every day, asking if he'd called the clinic. She bugged him until he was quite perturbed with her. Every day he had to make up some excuse: he was too busy to call, the results weren't back yet, the line was busy.

Finally, it was time for him to be released from the hospital. Bill, Elizabeth, and Luellen went to pick him up and deliver him to a house where he had rented himself a room. Luellen asked him about his HIV results, and he told her he had called the clinic and he was negative. It wasn't until eighteen months later that he admitted he had never gone back for the results.

Once out of rehab, Nick seemed to adjust to his new life and his newfound sobriety remarkably well. He contacted Melanie, and they decided they were better off without each other. "I'll always love her," he told his mother, "but we hurt each other too much."

Nick was relieved to be off drugs. He was happier and calmer than he had been in years. His relationships with his family and friends were improving. He and his father, a recovering alcoholic, attended twelve-step meetings together. He got back into a band with his old friends, and after a while he moved in with his friend Daveman, got a job, and seemed at long last to begin to take responsibility for himself.

A friend of Alex's had been interested in Nick while he was in the rehab, but when he got out, that relationship just sort of fizzled away. For the first time in many years, Nick stopped dating.

"Whatever happened to that girl who used to visit you at the rehab?" his mother asked him one day.

"Nothing." Nick was used to his mother always butting her nose into his business. Sometimes it upset him, but just now he felt warmed by her concern. "She lives in San Francisco, and she's going back east for college. We're just friends," he said.

"Are you seeing anybody else?"

"No, I need to take a break from dating." Nick could see his mother looked puzzled. "Listen, I've had enough sex to last a lifetime. I don't need any more, not right now." He stopped and looked up at her and smiled. "Don't worry, Mom, I'll date again when the time is right. Right now, I just need to take care of myself."

Nick tried not to think about whether or not he was HIV positive after he was released from the hospital, but even in his state of denial, he was afraid he might have it. He didn't want to infect anybody, so he avoided relationships that might develop into sexual relationships. Like so many others who know they are infected, or fear they are, he tried very hard to repress that information, to pretend it wasn't there. The mind is a powerful tool. If you tell yourself something isn't so, soon you come to believe it yourself. Nick succeeded in repressing the information fully. It became a nonissue for him. It didn't exist.

In September 1990, Nicolas decided to return to school and enrolled at DeAnza College. It was there he met Kim. She was the editor of the school paper, and he joined the staff of writers.

"She's not the prettiest girl I ever dated," he told his mother, "but she has a look about her that I really like. And she is so intelligent. She has one of the finest minds of anyone I've ever met."

Nick was attracted to Kim the first moment he saw her. He had to coax her a little before she was willing to make the big step of moving in together. "What have you got to lose?" Nick asked her. "If it doesn't work out, I'll just move out. I'll move out as soon as you say."

And so, Nick moved in with Kim. They had a lot in common, their writing, their odd way of dressing, their interest in literature, art, and music. Nick knew how to cook and was appalled that Kim often ate cold soup out of the can. He took great delight in preparing hearty meals for his newfound love. For Christmas, Kim bought Nick a custom Telecaster guitar. It was the most wonderful gift anyone had ever given him. He gave her a necklace that he found at a hippie shop.

Beneath this happy life that Nick was trying to create for himself was the two-edged sword protecting him from fearful reality. Yet, all the denial and all the lies couldn't keep the virus from doing its damage, and eventually the truth declared itself so loudly that it simply could not be denied any longer.

Six months after they met, Nick and Kim were facing the biggest challenge of their lives, AIDS.

When AIDS first entered the American psyche, the United States, under the Reagan Administration, abdicated its position of leadership because the disease was perceived to be a "gay" phenomenon. This notion was held because in the United States and Canada, AIDS primarily struck homosexual males. Never mind that in other parts of the world it was a heterosexual epidemic. That did not register with those who made policy and granted research funds. Gays were expendable. To combat the disease gays had to rally their own forces. They were forced by circumstance — as Nick discovered — to care for their own.

Even today when we know better, HIV/AIDS still carries the homosexual stigma. In spite of the fact that the number of HIV-positive teens in the United States *doubles* every 14 months, HIV/AIDS funding for research and education are under constant attack. (Karen Ocamb, "Gay and Lesbian Youth Emerge from Generational Shadows," *Gay & Lesbian Times*, August 10, 1995, p. 42).

CHAPTER FOUR

The Adjustment Begins

AIDS is the leading cause of death among Americans between the ages of twenty-five and forty-four. It is the sixth leading cause of death among fifteen- to twenty-four year olds in the United States. Worldwide, 3,000 women a day become HIV infected and 500 women die each day of AIDS. By the year 2000, between thirty and forty million men, women, and children will have been infected with HIV.

The statistics are staggering, but they don't tell the whole story. It is easier to hear the numbers than it is to comprehend what it is like to have AIDS. Nick was beginning to find out what it was like to have AIDS and how it affected every part of his life. He was beginning to make the adjustment from being a carefree young man with his whole life ahead of him to being a PWA (person with AIDS).

Several days after Nick came home from the hospital, he became so sick that he could not eat or sleep. He began to present symptoms of pancreatitis, which is sometimes caused by pentamadin. His doctor wanted him tested and ordered Nick to the emergency room. Luellen helped him into the car and they began the forty-five-minute trip to the hospital. On the way they talked.

"Nick, I truly wish that I was the one who was sick instead of you," his mother said.

"No you don't, Mom. Nobody would want to have what I have." He knew his mother was trying to be nice, but she couldn't be serious.

"I know it sounds patronizing," she said, "but it is true. I would do anything, if it were me instead of you."

"You don't know what you're saying. No one would want this virus."

Nick was watching his mother as she watched the road. "Yes, I do," she said. "For three reasons. First, I'm older than you. I've lived my life, or most of it. But you're only twenty-one; you still have your whole life ahead of you."

"That's crazy, Mom," he said. "You're only forty-one. You still have your whole life ahead of you, too."

"Second, I've had a lot of time to do all my spiritual research and to find myself. I know who I am, I've found my higher power, and I know where I'm going when I die. You are just beginning the journey. It takes time to discover who you are and who your God is. You need that time; I don't."

"Don't worry, I'll figure it out before my time is up." Nick was beginning to become impatient with the conversation.

"And finally, it is a far, far easier thing to die myself than to have to bury my own child."

Nick gazed out the car window, contemplating what his mother had just said. He was moved. After a few seconds, he looked at her. "That, I believe, is true," he said.

Nick discovered that even if one is well, a trip to a county hospital can make one sick. The first thing Nick and Luellen had to do when they got to the hospital was wait. They waited for more than three hours. Nick was feeling sicker and sicker by the moment. He didn't want to complain because that would make his mother worry and become impatient. He didn't like it when his mother worried or became impatient.

He tried to concentrate on not feeling sick, but finally he collapsed. Luellen stood in the dimly lit hallway with Nick crumpled at her feet. He heard his mother yell, "Help, my son has AIDS, please help." Normally, he would have been embarrassed at his mother making such a scene, but just then he was too sick to care.

Her yelling worked. From out of nowhere and everywhere nurses, doctors, and orderlies came running. They picked Nick up, put him in a wheelchair, escorted them to the triage nurse, and instructed her to give Nick the next bed in the emergency room.

The nurse smiled and nodded, put Nick in a bed, and promptly forgot about him.

By 7 P.M., Nick was starving. He told his mother he was sure if he could eat something he'd feel better. Luellen asked a nurse if she could get Nick a sandwich, explaining he hadn't eaten all day. The nurse was eating a Snickers bar. With her mouth full, she said Nick could not have anything to eat because if he had pancreatitis, eating would make him throw up.

Nick became more fidgety by the minute. When he heard he couldn't have any food, that was enough. He got up from the bed and pulled the heart monitor wires off his chest. He apologized to the nurse and told her very calmly that he was leaving. "Let's go to the deli across the street," he said to his mother.

"Okay," she said. "If you throw up, I can always bring you back."

"Yeah," he said, as they walked out of the emergency room.

He ate a Reuben sandwich, a large order of fries, and drank two cokes. Suddenly, he felt much better. When they got home, he ate two bowls of ice cream. And he didn't throw up. He concluded that he did not have pancreatitis.

After two weeks of convalescing at his parents' house, Nick went home to Pacifica with Kim. It was a huge relief to him to be free of his parents' hovering care, and it was wonderful to be back with Kim in their own place. Shortly after settling into their new home, Nick had his first appointment at the infectious disease clinic and was assigned a new doctor.

His CD4 cell count was 124. The CD4 count is the barometer by which the extent of HIV infection is measured. CD4 cells are a type of white blood cell whose job is to tell the other white cells what to do when there is an intruder in the body. HIV attaches itself to these cells and destroys them. Without sufficient CD4 cells, the other cells have no direction and cannot fight infection effectively. A normal CD4 count is 1000 or higher.

The virus had also attacked his nervous system, causing a condition called neuropathy that was in his feet and spreading into his legs. His feet were sensitive to touch, and the burning sensations were often so intense that he used ice to relieve the discomfort. He took dapsone to prevent a reoccurrence of pneumocystic pneumonia and was started on AZT.

Nick settled into his routine. He and Kim and the rest of his family tried to get on with their lives. Only now, Nick's life was significantly different from what it had ever been before. Now it was full of trips to the doctor, medications, tests, and discomfort.

On June 25, Nick had his first appointment with the third new doctor, Dr. Donald Polanski, a leading authority in AIDS research and treatment. Dr. Polanski did not take Medi-Cal patients in his private practice, but he decided to make an exception in Nick's case. (Medi-Cal is the federally funded health insurance program for poor people in California.) Nick was very pleased that the doctor was impressed enough with him to give him preferential treatment.

Dr. Polanski sent Nicolas to a community research project to see if he could be included in their project. Nick needed to be tested for mycobacterium avium intracellulare (MAI), a rare kind of tuberculosis that many people with AIDS get. Medi-Cal didn't cover that test, but this particular test was part of the screening process for getting into the research study. Nick's doctor recommended him to be a part of the research project so that Nick could get tests and treatment that he wouldn't be able to get otherwise.

Nick was adamant that he should still live his life and do the things he would have been doing if he had not been sick. He was in a band called "soulburning flashes," which now met at his house in Pacifica to practice. Practices were different than they had been before. Sometimes, Nick did the whole practice in bed, with the rest of the band gathered around his bedroom.

He and Kim and some of their friends decided to produce a concert to raise money for *Static*, a newsmagazine they had been publishing for about six months. Nick was excited about this project, and he spent a lot of time working on it. He was very proud that he had been able to contribute so much, in spite of his illness. He invited his parents to come to the concert.

Nick and Kim and a few other people were standing outside the club where the concert was to be held when he saw his parents coming toward him. Smiling broadly, Nick walked up the street to meet his parents.

"Mom, Dad!" he exclaimed. "You came."

"Well, of course we came," Luellen said. "We wouldn't have missed it."

"Come on, I want you to meet Kim's parents."

Nick made the introductions, and they all went into the shabby, dark nightclub. In one corner, a table had been set up and some of Kim's and Nick's friends were selling T-shirts that Nick had designed for the occasion. They were also giving away copies of *Static*.

After a few minutes, Nick and the other members of his band took the stage. Nick was wearing black leggings, a T-shirt, and a secondhand sport jacket festooned with safety pins and masking tape. He picked up his Telecaster and his band began to play. All of the songs were written by Nick, and he sang the lead to most of them.

His on-stage persona was mature and confident. He felt good. This was what he loved to do and it showed. His singing was loud and strong. For a few moments, he could forget he had AIDS and just be himself, the Nickman. It was impossible to detect, as he pranced around the stage, that only a few weeks before he had been in the hospital hooked up to oxygen, or that even as he was infecting the audience with his own brand of musical excitement, the infection in his body was slowly sucking his life away.

The deadly disease would not be forgotten for long, however. Toward the end of July, Nick got the news that his CD4 count had dropped to 91. He became anemic and was feeling very run-down. He was tired of fighting to be normal and he needed a rest, so he and Kim went to his parents' house for a few days. Kim and Elizabeth spent the time doing Nick's and Kim's laundry. Nick napped and ate.

Nick regained some of his strength at home and began to write an article for *Static* on what his experiences with AIDS were like. When he had first been diagnosed, he hadn't wanted anyone to know he was sick, but now he was beginning to think that he should share his story. He had also realized that there were people in his life whom he had to tell. One of those people was Melanie.

It was a very difficult thing for him to do, because he was afraid that he might have infected her. One day while he was at his mother's, he told his mom about the encounter with Melanie. They were sitting in the backyard. "Mom, I called Melanie a couple of weeks ago," he said. "I needed to tell her about my situation so that she could get tested."

"How did it go?" his mom asked.

"I was really nervous about it," he said, "but it went okay. I just told her I needed to see her, and she said that would be okay. Kim and I took her out to lunch in San Francisco. I just

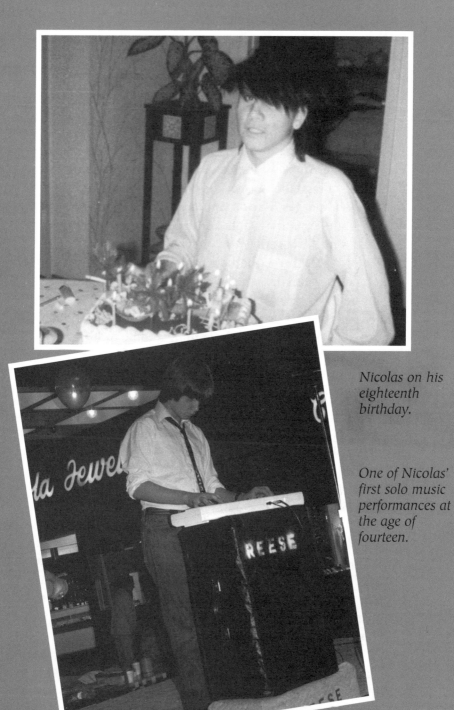

Nicolas on his
eighteenth
birthday.

One of Nicolas'
first solo music
performances at
the age of
fourteen.

told her I had AIDS and she was okay about it. She said she would get tested right away and let me know." Nick stopped to rest for a while. "She was very concerned about me, but I told her I'm fine, and not to worry. She was glad I told her."

"I'm really proud of you for doing that. I know it took a lot of courage," said Luellen.

"Courage doesn't have anything to do with it. I had to tell her, that's all. Anyway, she called the other day. She's negative. That's a big relief to me. Kim's negative, too. Her doctor said she should get tested every six months while she lives with me, but her father wants her to get tested every month."

Nick was discovering that having AIDS is an up-and-down kind of thing, both emotionally and physically. Sometimes he felt cool, and sometimes he felt lousy. He was dealing with his anger, his guilt, and trying to adjust to all the changes in his life and in his body. Sometimes, though, he just wanted to forget about the whole thing and be ordinary.

The last morning he was home, he woke up at six-thirty. Bill had already left for work and Luellen was in bed doing the crossword puzzle in the morning paper when he came into the room.

"I'm tired of watching Kim sleep," he said as he climbed into bed with his mother just like he used to do when he was little. He just wanted to be normal. He wanted to be Nick, not a person with AIDS. For a few minutes while he and his mother sat in bed and talked about other things, he almost felt normal.

In September, the results of Nick's MAI test finally came back and were negative. His band, soulburning flashes, released a tape of six songs written by Nick and it was getting air play on several of the local radio stations, as well as selling in record shops. Nick was pleased when Elizabeth told him how excited she was because the bookstore at her college was also selling the tape. A lot of her friends were buying it and saying to her, "Aren't you Nick Trevor's sister?"

It was a few days later, during a simple trip to San

Francisco that Nick quietly slipped into the realization that he really did have AIDS and that it was not going to go away. That morning, Kim went to San Francisco. Nick was to take the bus and the BART train into the city to meet her that afternoon. He took the bus to the BART station and, true to form, when he got there, he realized he did not have enough money to buy a BART ticket, nor did he have enough to take another bus back home to get more funds.

He decided to hang around the BART station until he saw someone who looked gay so he could ask him if he could borrow the fare for the BART. He felt it would be foolhardy for someone who looked like him to ask anyone other than a gay person for assistance. He was now painfully aware of the fact that he looked like he had AIDS and many people were not as accepting as the gay population.

Shortly, Nick saw a well-dressed, thirty-something businessman carrying a briefcase. He approached the man and said, "Excuse me, sir."

The man turned around and said, "Nick, isn't it?" The man was in an HIV-positive support group Nick had attended one time. "How are you doing?" the man asked.

Nick felt relieved, almost happy that he had found one of his own kind. He explained his predicament to the gentleman. The man bought Nick a BART ticket and two candy bars. He got on the BART train with Nick and rode with him to his stop. Nick felt a camaraderie with this man, and it felt comfortable. He was now a member of a special group of extraordinary people fighting an extraordinary battle. The man got off the BART train with Nick and waited with him until Kim arrived. Nick knew this was the kind of thing people with HIV did for each other. They took care of each other. They had to.

One of the problems of any disease is that the general public "cocoons," protecting itself through ignorance of the disease itself and those afflicted with it. We may ask how others are out of a cordial politeness. But the fact is, most of us don't want to hear unpleasantdetails.

It was no different with AIDS. But if ignorance is bliss, then the general public was severely shaken when All-American Rock Hudson was diagnosed with AIDS. Until then, AIDS had been relatively anonymous and very few people knew anyone with the disease. Suddenly, AIDS had a face. But it was an old face. It was a gay face. Nick and Kim provide us with two young faces, each dealing with HIV/AIDS in different ways.

CHAPTER FIVE

Nick and Kim Speak

Nick's story about AIDS was finally finished and became the center point of an issue of *Static* devoted to the AIDS epidemic. "On Being Poor, Being Alive and Having AIDS" by Nicolas J. Trevor was printed in the September/ October 1991 issue. In the prolog, he referred to a time when he was raped. When he was diagnosed with AIDS, he suspected that the rape may have been the occasion when he contracted HIV. He began to realize, however, that he had engaged in all the at-risk behaviors available to him and was in fact never sure how or when he was infected.

I'm still breathing. When it comes right down to it, I am still breathing.

I'm staring out the window quite a bit these days, I'm not sure what I'm looking for, so, I'm just looking, and I notice that I'm still breathing.

I sit back and think back across the years of my life. The camera pans, and then zooms in on a fifteen-year-

old boy. Tears rolling down his face, screaming at the top of his lungs, he's leaving home.

A seventeen-year-old boy arguing with an art professor, the professors never knew what they were talking about, or so our character thought.

A nineteen-year-old boy is . . . in one of those 10-dollar-a-night hotels on Polk Street . . . tears streaming again . . .

Sometimes I don't want to know who this boy is, but I do. A twenty-one-year-old man is lying in a hospital bed, the doctor comes in and puts her hand on the man's leg, "Well, it's AIDS . . . "

Again the tears begin to roll.

I'm staring out the window a lot these days.

I'm still breathing.

Being Alive

by Nicholas J. Trevor

So, I wake up in a hospital bed with an oxygen hose in my face and a little plastic doohickie between my legs to pee in. My closest friends surround me like I was some sort of holy ghost. I've just been diagnosed with full-blown AIDS.

It's sort of funny. In high school, saying someone was gay was a derogatory remark used on people who looked different or didn't play football. Needless to say, the rumors abounded. With the rumors (some of which may have been true some of the time) came the AIDS jokes. Even among friends, I would jest about AIDS, "Say there, when ya gonna finally shake that nasty AIDS bug?" How ironic.

That was a different time.

Upon being discharged from the county hospital, I quit my job, went on disability and began to do battle with symptoms, AZT (AZT is an antiviral drug that slows down the reproduction of the virus. The side effects of AZT are unpleasant to say the least) and everyone else's philosophy on how I should handle my life.

Ugh! So what does everyone expect? Do I have to take AZT, do yoga, listen to Louise Hay's meditation tapes telling me that AIDS is both a challenge and a gift? No way. AIDS is not a challenge and a gift. Maybe a challenging pain in the ass, but not a gift. Do I have to have my blood boiled, drawn, tested and counted? Or do I take mounds of Chinese herbs and spend my Wednesday afternoons on the acupuncturist's table? I'm no fucking victim.

I've been real lucky, though. At least I've had friends to tell me how to run my life. So many people with AIDS go through life alone. For the life of me, I just don't know how anyone could handle this alone, but they do.

After some procrastination, I decided to check out some of the PWA support groups in the Bay Area. I heard a lot of what I expected, "We're all victims! What do we do?" (No, it wasn't that bad, but the idea was evident enough to turn me off.) I now think that support groups can be very beneficial to those newly diagnosed, but as I grow in my illness, I find more support from those I love and live with.

Are we not free? Or are we AIDS victims dying of AIDS? I prefer to look at it as living with AIDS. Which brings up an interesting point. Get ready folks for a shocker: AIDS is not 100 percent fatal. No shit!

It blew me away when I first heard it. You see, there are alive today many people (mostly men, unfortunately) who were diagnosed as early as 1978 who are still alive and kickin'. Of course these numbers are comparatively small but they do exist and that gives me hope. The statistics are there, and you know how the American people love statistics. Personally, I despise statistics.

Statistics are hard to ignore, and though I try not to pay heed, it's really hard when you see numbers like 80 percent of males live 2 to 4 years and 99 percent of females 12 to 18 months, and then the doctors tell us that no one likes to give any sort of prognosis. Fifty percent of all people with AIDS (PWAs) with T-cell counts (T-cells instruct the immune system what to attack. The HIV virus destroys these cells.) below 50 contract CMV retinitis and go blind. CMV retinitis is an inflammation in the retina caused by cytomegalovirus, a microbe which causes many different infections.

I'm still alive, and I'm still breathing, regardless of the statistical data.

Being Poor

Then there's the money. Big pain. I checked myself into the emergency room at Santa Clara Valley Medical Center on April 22, but I had been deathly ill since January and feeling very under the weather for nearly a year. Like most other poor folk, I had no medical insurance to speak of, so I sat around for months and months getting sicker and sicker. Finally the time came when I absolutely had to do something about my condition. I was horrified for two reasons: I didn't have a dime to my name, and I was afraid of what the diagnosis might be.

After a lot of beating around the bush I was finally brought to the emergency room. Literally dragged in on the shoulders of the woman I love . . . I collapsed at the E.R.'s triage counter. What a mess. There I was propped up against one of the couches in a huge waiting room with a hundred other sick dying poor folk.

Looking around the room was like surveying all the world's damned, waiting and moaning until the nicely dressed nurse walks through the heavy door and blurts out a name. Like handing out salvation at the gates of purgatory, and that's glamorizing it all.

Soon, my name was called, and I was brought to the intake clerk who needed to ask me some questions about my income. What income? No insurance. No Medi-Cal. No money. No reason to live, might as well box me up and ship me right out then and there.

But this was a county hospital, with a tiny little sign that read, "No person shall be denied treatment due to lack of funds," and I sure as hell had a lack of funds.

All the questions . . .

"Do you own any real property? Do you own any stocks or bonds?"

"Cough."

"Do you have life insurance? Are you the benefactor of any trusts or accounts?"

Meanwhile, I'm hacking and heaving and on the verge of passing out.

"Do you have any valuables?"

"Cough."

"Do you have any jewelry?"

This one was the real killer: "Do you own any musical instruments?" Yikes! I do have a couple of guitars. I was not about to declare them. So I lied. Ha!

After the third degree designed to ascertain the value of my being, I was asked to sign a form stating that the hospital was not responsible for anything in my possession at the time of admission that might become lost, stolen or damaged.

Finally, I was told that the hospital has a program called "Ability to Pay."

However to apply for the Ability to Pay program, you must also apply for Medi-Cal. Mountains of paperwork, legalese and dollar sign bullcrap, and all I want to know is WHY I CAN'T BREATHE!

Finally, after signing away my life to the county, I was told that I could, at last, go back to the waiting room and wait some more. Soon I was brought to the nurse's desk where they would decide how much longer I should wait before I could get a table in the E.R. More questions.

"Can you breathe?'

"Are there any white patches in your mouth?"

And then the killer, "Are you HIV-positive?"

I didn't know what to say.

The nurse looks at me with a knowing eye and puts my file in the urgent bin. Eventually, I was seen.

It's the same old story, it's a county hospital just like any other county hospital in any major urban area. One gets the feeling that one is being herded like cattle on account of their finances.

It's a double-edged sword with AIDS. In the mid-'80s there was a lot of hysteria surrounding the fact that the over-whelming majority of Americans thought that people with AIDS were out-and-out deviants. A disease to get rid of all them "fags and junkies," and so many fags and junkies are poor. Hence the bitter AIDS stigma.

Directly across the street from the county's E.R. is the I.C.H. clinic where the county's indigent PWA population is treated. At one of my numerous visits to the E.R., I was con-fronted by some bitchy nurse who looked at me and said, "HIV-positive! Why aren't you across the street with the rest of them?" The rest of them? What the hell is this? So, in the eyes of this nurse, I'm just a "THEM."

The poor and HIV-infected confront an awful lot of barri-ers, but there are many organizations that do everything from feed and clothe PWAs to taking them out to dinner and a movie. There's even some organizations that will clean your kitchen and go to the grocery store for you. As long as you are one of "THEM."

Even with all the amazing support available to PWAs, it's still pretty tough trying to get by on a social security budget with medical costs approaching the $50,000 mark. AZT alone costs around $1,500 a month, not to mention nursing costs, hospital costs, and the cost of stress taxing the soul. Fortunately, for me, my Medi-Cal was approved through my social security program, and they gave me four stickers a month to take care of whatever medical expenses. . . . . There's a trick that people on Medi-Cal have devised. If the clerk taking your payment is cool, you can ask her to photocopy your sticker and use that, it works for billing and Medi-Cal never seems to mind. The only thing is convincing the clerk to go for it. Doctors usually will, pharmacists usually don't.

Having AIDS

So many of my attitudes have changed, so much of my lifestyle has changed, but I'm still the same old guy. I love to stay up all night, play loud music, read strange literature, and take long drives down the coast. But things are different. Strangely enough, my sex life has picked up. I had more hanky-panky than I ever thought was possible for a really sick dude.

I remember reading a pamphlet written by Dan Turner, cofounder of the San Francisco AIDS Foundation. I read the first thing you should do is quit your job, go on disability, don't do anything you don't enjoy, do the things you love.

Some of the things I hate are some of the things my doctors think I should be doing. AZT for instance has been a big dilemma for me. I was first prescribed AZT in May, when I was still getting over my bout with pneumocystis carinii pneumonia. (One of the many opportunistic infections. In the past it was 100 percent fatal, but now is easily treatable with sulfa and other kinds of drugs.) I was constantly feeling shitty, but I persevered and stayed with the stuff until August when my doctor doubled the dose. I tried my best, really I did, but as I write this in mid-September, I haven't taken any all month. I'm not sure how much it's helping me feel better to know that I'm not swallowing poison five times a day, even if it does work.

My latest fling has been with Eastern medicine, Chinese herbs and acupuncture. I've got this herbalist who has concocted a formula that just might take care of some of the worst symptoms I've been having: energy loss, high fevers and peripheral neuropathy (also called the Polynesian Fire Walk, numbness and painful burning sensations in the hands and feet). It's another irony of sorts — I hated having to take five doses of AZT every day, so now I take twenty-eight herbal pills every day in addition to numerous vitamins and an experimental drug.

One of the things PWAs are occasionally asked to do is to take part in double blind/placebo drug trials. This is where neither the patient nor the health care workers know who's getting the real stuff. So, I'm taking this experimental drug and it works out for the better. In exchange for my precious time and energy, they do all of my blood work, and work with my doctor taking a whole lot of the load off of his back.

All in all, I've enjoyed doing the drug trial. My health care worker is HIV-positive himself, I find that very comforting considering all the recent hoopla about whether or not doctors should be allowed to have AIDS and all that. As a matter of fact, my health care worker at the clinic referred me to the Chinese herbalist, so everything is sort of interconnected.

So, where do we go from here? Forward. I'm not afraid, I'm not a total emotionless machine, either. I get my bad days and my much worse than bad days. Recently, I've actually come to the realization that it's okay to be sad. Feel the sadness and then carry on. I try not to get carried away with the negativity, but it is there. Some of my friends say that I can get pretty gloomy, maybe even depressed. When I asked my doctor about seeing a shrink, he smiled and said that I didn't strike him as the type that needed a shrink. Hmmm.

So, I'm staring out the window a lot these days. I don't even care if I don't know exactly what I'm looking for, because I'm making the best of it. I'm with the ones that I love. I do the things that I love. And I'm still breathing.

In the same issue of *Static,* the following article by Kim Hecht, the woman Nick loved, also appeared.

A Nation of Ostriches

by Kim Hecht

Late at night when all the lights in the house are off and I can't sleep because I'm lying in bed, listening for hitches in Nicolas' breathing, hoping that it's not the return of the pneumonia that landed Nick in the hospital and almost killed him, the pneumonia that turned out to be AIDS related, I start to think. How different our little family has become from everyone else's. We don't think like other people anymore. We think in life and death terms, and there is very little planning ahead, because it is all too possible tomorrow might never come.

Late in those nights, when the leaves rustle against the windows, and Nick's body grows hot from another fever, I suddenly realize that I'm nineteen years old but I feel like I'm one hundred. I can no longer relate to the people I went to high school with four years ago.

Then I was just another girl. Now, to most of them, I'm someone they might read about in Newsweek. *The goals we shared have lost meaning — finishing college doesn't seem that important anymore, nor does a career or partying or any of the things that we most often talked about. Nicolas and I walk in a place most of them know nothing of, where death is never far away from our thoughts.*

I know that I am in a different world from most people now. But why? Of course any fatal illness is frightening and hard for healthy people to relate to. But there is a core of denial and repulsion with AIDS that does not exist for people with terminal lung cancer or Lou Gehrig's disease.

What I eventually realized is that for the majority of people, despite the endless media depictions, AIDS does not have a human face. They are separated from people with AIDS by an emotional barrier of otherness. To put it bluntly, people with AIDS are faggots and drug addicts, and therefore less than human.

The article "The Implicated and the Immune" by Richard Goldstein, from the book *A Disease of Society*, explains this very well. "AIDS," he writes, "more than even other sexually transmitted diseases, has seemed to 'select' its victims from among previously defined groups: at first, homosexuals and IV-drug users; and more recently, women of color and their children." It is this quality of selectiveness, he says, that "has made it possible for mass culture to assume the perspective of a 'witness' to AIDS who also stands outside it."

So although the bombardment by the news media means that anyone who gets a newspaper or has a radio is aware of AIDS, its severity, and its consequences, few people outside of the gay community have any deep emotional response to the disease. AIDS, when it comes right down to it, is still an "Us-versus-Them" disease. This fear and feeling of separation has allowed people to suggest such inhumane measures as quarantining, long after methods of transmission were understood. A Blendon and Donelan survey showed that in 1988, 30 percent of Americans still supported some sort of quarantine for people with the HIV virus in their blood.

I first started noticing this "witness" tone a few weeks after Nicolas was diagnosed. I was, of course, reading everything I could get my hands on about AIDS. As I came to accept living with a person with AIDS (PWA), it became harder to move from the literature of the AIDS programs, or the gay community, to the mainstream media, where everyone with AIDS is an AIDS VICTIM, and is DYING TRAGICALLY. The media seems to assume anyone with AIDS should thereafter be defined by their illness.

I find this Us-versus-Them or "witness" tone taken in the major publications appalling. Television and movies, where most people get their insight into other peoples' lives, continues to perpetuate and reinforce old stereotypes.

According to prime time, we live in a society where gays, drug users, and sick people are Other. Thus we can pity them, the newspapers whisper, but we can't relate to them. Their difficulties, it seems, are no closer to our hearts than those of the Kurds in Iraq. Further, maybe. We (or at least so the media tells us) are the healthy, young, beautiful (mostly white) people. And that's the way we should want it to stay.

The more I observe from my new–found position as one of Them, the more I realize that we are a society that wishes to remain safe, even if safety is only illusory. No one escapes death and illness; suffering and misfortune are forever only a roll of the dice away. But even death is so martinized, santized, and hidden away by our consumer-oriented culture that it is no longer considered something we have to suffer, if we eat enough wheat germ.

We are a nation of people that has come to believe that death is something unnatural and we don't want to be reminded that it is going to happen to us. On every doctor's waiting room table is a copy of *Longevity Magazine*, with beautiful, fit models telling us that if we cut down on our cholesterol, if we exercise and eat right, we will never die. We want to believe it so badly that we adopt a selective blindness.

People Magazine publishes a special edition every so often entitled "The 50 Most Beautiful People in the World." The Spring 1991 edition contained an editorial by Richard Lacayo that gives an interesting look into America's views on the subjects of beauty and living forever. "As we said earlier," he writes, "we're always on the lookout for beauty because it says things we can't express in words. One of those things is our desire to live forever. And in their way, Great Looking People, kindle our hopes for eternity."

What does that say about how a society will react to the man whose face is covered with the purple blotches of kaposi's sarcoma (a cancer that often strikes PWAs)? Who is going to be able to feel good around him? Who is going to want to be around him? His very presence will have the opposite effect from that Great Looking Person's reminding us of the possibility of death, and so we separate ourselves from him, not just physically, but by constructing an invisible barrier of otherness.

People even seem to be afraid that the very presence of the ill will infect them. For instance, an issue of Newsweek this spring reported that many people survive cancer with paid sick leave from their workplaces only to get fired when they return because their employers don't want to be near someone who had cancer, who would be a reminder of their own mortality. Now multiply that times 10 for any PWA.

David Wojnarowicz, a gay artist and author with AIDS, writes that people ". . . feel quite safe from any terrible event or problem such as homelessness or AIDS or nonexistent medical care or rampant crime or hunger or unemployment or racism or sexism simply because they go to sleep every night in a house or apartment or dormitory whose clean walls or regular structures of repeated daily routines provide them with a feeling of safety that never gets intruded upon by the events outside."

This ability to feel safe in the face of terrible situations is having desperate consequences. It is leading to a society where people ignore problems. Sure, there is compassion. But it is far too often compassion without action. Helping others has become the occasional hobby of the rich, rather than a way of life for everyone. There has to be an incentive, like nine hours of big-name bands. Compassionate attendance at Live-Aid, uh huh.

A phrase of the generals is "divide and conquer." This country (and others) is doing this to itself. If America collaps-

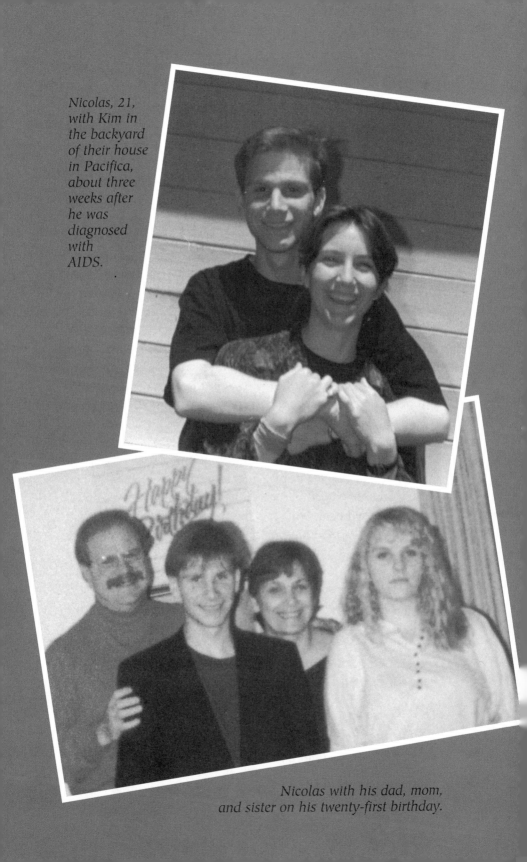

Nicolas, 21, with Kim in the backyard of their house in Pacifica, about three weeks after he was diagnosed with AIDS.

Nicolas with his dad, mom, and sister on his twenty-first birthday.

es, whether because of garbage buildup, global warming or nuclear war, it will most likely be because it was always the problem of the "other guy." If we just ignore him, the problem will go away, thinks your average American, who these days is better represented by the ostrich than the eagle.

And getting back to the idea of compassion — I have often heard it suggested that AIDS will never be the enormous threat to the heterosexual population that experts now predict, but that creating hysteria about possible infection was, however, the only way to get the straight population to do anything about AIDS.

Well, I'll let the experts argue about infection vectors and what not. But I do know that at last report there were 118,000 deaths* from AIDS in America ALONE. That's more than twice as many as the number of American soldiers killed in Vietnam. And I suggest that if this seems less meaningful to you because only maybe 6 percent were confirmed totally and completely heterosexual, non-drug using, and not from Haiti, then you are pretty cold.

Unfortunately, for a lot of people it still does make a difference, like all the people who laugh their guts out when comedian Sam Kinison asserts that gay men spread lies about the need to use condoms in order to repress the heterosexual libido, and jokes about HIV being caused by gay men's propensity for "screwing monkeys."

The federal government is not overflowing with compassion, either. In case you think it is, let's try a little comparison here. The defense budget for 1990 ran something along the line of 200 billion dollars. For AIDS there was the Ryan White Bill, which released, at long last, emergency monies of about 200 million to go to desperately needy hospitals and groups. It was then cut to 88 million, of which only 44 million ever

---

* *By 1995, more than 300,000 people had died of AIDS in the U. S. and more than 3,000,000 worldwide.*

saw the light of day. Is there any clearer message that people with AIDS are expendable?

Or, if this comparison seems a little unfair (after all, this is defense for the whole country, and these are only a couple of sick people), try comparing expenditures on toxic shock syndrome, or legionnaires' disease. In both cases, millions and millions were immediately spent to find the cause of diseases hurting only a few isolated people. It took months, and several hundred deaths, before recognition was given to AIDS, let alone funding.

So I think I have a pretty good basis when I say that everyday compassion is necessary. No one is going to take care of our problems for us and we can't consider buying a ticket to Live-Aid as enough anymore. There can be no more "I'll pay attention to that when I have more time, when I'm making 30k a year." We have to do something now, something real. We have to face our fears and try to create a better reality, not hide from it. Death may be inevitable, but a painful life is not. I challenge you to do something now. And if we can't act together to save our own, then maybe we deserve whatever plagues we get.

So as I lie in bed late at night and listen to Nicolas coughing, I want in your minds to be the thought that Nicolas' favorite ice cream is Rainforest Crunch. That when he sleeps he curls up on his side. That he calls our kitten M.C. Kitty and makes up raps for it. That in the third month I knew him he cleaned my entire apartment for me while I was at school and left a love poem on the bed which was so beautiful that I cried. I want you to think about it all and say Nicolas is expendable. That he is one of Them.

As AIDS became a media topic worthy of mainstream consideration, many conservative religious leaders, televangelists, and politicians saw it as a means to fill coffers and ballot boxes. Instead of offering Christian compassion and political support for research funding, these groups pointed the finger of blame. In a fiery speech before the 1992 Republican National Convention, Patrick Buchanan, the darling of the religious right, charged that AIDS was Nature's retribution for homosexuality (Larry Dane Brimner, *Being Different: Lambda Youths Speak Out*, (Danbury, Conn.: Franklin Watts), p. 115). His comments may have bolstered his political clout among the Christian Coalition and other conservative, political/religious organizations, but they severely stung families grappling with the disease. Nothing seemed more accusatory, more anti-Christian, however, than the actions of Philadelphia's Bishop Nathan Giddings, who posted a sign on the front of his church reading ". . . to join you must have an AIDS test and it must come back Negative" (William R. Macklin, "Tiny Church Stirs Big Controversy," *San Diego Union-Tribune*, December 25, 1994, p. A-36).

Overcoming the Guilt

In the middle of October, Nick went to the doctor to get the latest lab results. The news was bad and disturbed Nick very much. He could see his agitated mood was distressing Kim, but he couldn't put his own mind to rest, let alone comfort her.

He was relieved when she suggested he call his mother, but was too downcast to respond. He watched as Kim picked up the phone and dialed Luellen.

Kim is a small girl, quiet and unassuming, but her petite looks and her subdued manner belied the strength of her character. Nick listened as she spoke to his mother, preparing her for the mood he was in. After a few minutes, she handed the phone to Nick.

"Mom, I didn't get good news at the doctor's today." He was dazed. "My CD4 count is down to 48. It's falling fast."

"This isn't good news, but it's not the worst news, either," his mother said.

"I don't want to talk about it," Nick said.

Nick had stopped taking his AZT because it made him feel sick. Maybe that was the reason for this drop in the CD4 count, and maybe it was his attitude, which had lately become very negative. And maybe it was just the virus picking up steam.

Guilt is a heavy burden to carry. It can tire one out; it was exhausting Nick. He would try to push it out of his mind, and then, when he least expected it, it would come out of nowhere and shake his confidence, his self-esteem, making him angry and depressed.

While he had been at his mother's house soon after his diagnosis, Nick and his mom were sitting at the dining room table, talking. From beneath the calm surface he tried always to project, the anguish he was feeling began to bubble up uncontrollably.

"What's wrong?" Luellen asked him.

"What do you think is wrong?" he snapped. "I have AIDS."

"I meant is there something in particular that is bothering you?"

Nick studied his hands for a few seconds. He didn't quite want to say what he was feeling. He knew his mother was persistent and wouldn't let it drop, so he just spit it out. "A lot of people think people who have AIDS deserve it. I guess I'm thinking I deserve it."

"What, like AIDS is a punishment for doing bad things?" Luellen said.

"Well, I certainly did a lot of things that I shouldn't have done." Nick was beginning to understand that he had created his life.

"Yes, so?"

"If I hadn't done those things, I wouldn't be sick now."

"Maybe that's true, but there is a big difference between acquiring the results of having lived an at-risk lifestyle and deserving a terrible disease. Nobody deserves AIDS. You don't deserve AIDS. Do you think people who smoke deserve cancer? Do you think people who drink too much deserve cirrhosis of the liver?"

Nick shook his head. He wanted to believe what his mother was saying, but he wasn't quite convinced.

"Then why do you think you deserve AIDS?" Luellen continued." It's the same thing." She reached across the table and took Nick's hand. "You don't deserve AIDS."

He looked at her, his eyes pleading for an answer that would put his mind to rest, then he just shrugged. "Forget it, Mom."

At the urging of his doctor, Nick went back on the AZT. The drop in his CD4 count scared him, at least temporarily, into trying to take a little better care of himself. A few days later, his mom went up to Pacifica to visit him for the day. He was putting out the trash as she arrived. He dropped the bags into the can and saw his mother eyeing the beer cans and tequila bottles among the debris.

"Did you have a party?" she asked.

"No," he answered, perturbed that she was sounding like a mother. "Paul and Alex have been staying here and they drink."

"I hope you aren't drinking," Luellen said.

"Mom, I'm an adult, you know."

They went into the house. "I have some more news that is kind of bad," he said. "The doctor gave me morphine for the pain." He paused to see her reaction.

"If it helps with the pain, take it," Luellen said, "but try not to take too much."

"Mom, it's addictive."

"I know." She paused. "Isn't there something else the doctor could give you?"

"Nothing that works. Doctor Polanski says not to worry. He says there is no reason that I shouldn't be comfortable."

"Of course not," she said.

"You know they only give morphine to people who are going to be dead in a few weeks," he said quite matter-of factly.

"Yes, and I also know they have no idea how long you will live. All they can do is guess."

Nick nodded.

November 9, 1991, was Nick's twenty-second birthday. He didn't want to celebrate or even acknowledge his birthday. His parents offered to have a party and invite his family and Kim's, but he said no. They offered to take him and Kim out to dinner, but he said no. They finally offered to just come over and visit. He didn't like that idea either but relented and allowed them to come.

They arrived with a cake baked by Elizabeth, a card, and a gift. Nick was resting when his parents got there. Kim's mom and aunt were there sorting through Kim's stuff. Paul and Alex were visiting.

They all chatted for a while and ate Liz's cake. Then Nick had a burst of energy and said, "Where are you taking me?" He had been so adamant about not celebrating his birthday that it was a surprise to everyone. Nick remembered being invited to go out and now he wanted to go. So they went. The birthday had given him a brief respite from his guilt, the cake had given him some energy, and suddenly he wanted to get out of the house.

Nick and Kim and Nick's parents went to Japan Town and ate at a Japanese restaurant with tables that had electric hibachis, allowing the customers to cook their own food. Nick had a great time cooking his squid. They went to an Asian import shop and bought all kinds of little junk which can only be found in an Asian import shop. Nick bought a "people's" hat from China and a pocketknife. He loved pocketknives.

"This was a lot of fun," Nick said on the way home. He was beaming all over. "Today reminded me of when I was little and we'd do tourist things together as a family. Thanks a lot, you guys."

Two days later, he and Kim flew to New York and Philadelphia to visit some of his relatives and some of hers.

Nick wrote one of his rare letters to his folks while he was there.

November 13, 1991

Mom & Dad,

Well, here I am, having a blast. Real cold, but I'm doing fine.

I think I'm beginning to realize that I must be a New Yorker at heart. Everything I need seems to be right here.

I've been hanging out at N.Y.U. all day and elsewhere in Greenwich Village. I want to stay. But not to worry, I'm coming back. I still think S.F. is a little more me.

You know I was thinking back to a conversation we had a while back about where home is; 623 Browns Valley [the long time home of Nick's maternal grandparents] or 1088 Fillipelli [a recent home of Nick's family] or wherever. There were so many different places.

Now that I think about it, more than anywhere else I feel my home is San Francisco.

Although home is where the soul resides, physicality of places makes a difference.
I love you,

Be back soon,
Nick

While they were back East, Nick and Kim went to see the movie, *The Rapture*, a film about a woman with a dull job who is searching for more meaning to life than her hedonistic lifestyle provides. She turns to fundamentalist religious fanaticism and in the film ascends into heaven. Nick was so agitated by the movie that he called his mother from New York in the middle of the day. "I need to talk about this movie I just saw," he said. "I don't know why, but it really scared me."

The movie had affected him deeply. He was consumed with guilt over his past life. He was certain he was being punished and that his punishment would continue into the next life, which he was now beginning to think actually existed. He confessed to his mother he had been having terrorizing dreams in which people and things were always trying to destroy him.

"Mom, I've lived a bad life and now I'm getting what I deserve," he said.

"No, that's not true." Luellen tried to reassure him. "You've done a lot of things that you shouldn't have done, but you've also done a lot of good things, wonderful and kind things. You have not lived a bad life."

"Then why do I feel the way I do?" he pleaded.

"For most of your life, you've avoided the spiritual side of life, and now that you are faced with the ultimate test of having a disease that is most often fatal, you are forced to consider things that most people your age don't have to think about, and you are afraid."

Nick listened intently. He was desperate for answers. His mother continued. "You have all the answers you need within you, but you haven't bothered to look before. What you need to tell yourself is that God is a loving and merciful God. Try to relax and quiet your mind and then ask him for help."

They talked for an hour and by the end of the conversation he relaxed a little, but was still within the grotesque grip of guilt. The movie, the dreams, all were frightening to him. The fear of the unknown, the idea of being punished, all these things sat in his consciousness and worried him.

When he got home from the East, he was pleased to find a letter from his mother following up on the phone conversation they had had. In it, she picked up the thread of the conversation she and Nick had about death and guilt:

My first thought is this: If a person is coming from the position that he/she deserves a disease (or any "bad" situation), then it is most likely assured that that person will never recover from or overcome that disease/situation. Perhaps the context you've created is one of deserving AIDS and perhaps that unconscious supposition is what keeps you from taking your meds properly and caring for yourself more enthusiastically, and maybe that is why your disease is progressing more rapidly.

In any case, let's get rid of that supposition, now! You do not deserve this disease! Nobody does. Guilt is a very destructive waste of time and energy. Please forgive yourself for whatever it is you think you did that makes you feel you deserve AIDS.

It is as you say, really. You were experimenting, pushing the limits, testing yourself and life. That is what all young people do. Did you go a little farther than most go? Maybe. Do a lot of people go farther than you did? Absolutely. Did you make mistakes? Yes, but as a member of the human race, you are entitled to make mistakes, lots of them. Nothing you did deserves this disease. This disease is an unfair aberration that has attacked the human race in a way that is frightening and vicious. It calls us, all of us, to be the very best we can be, spiritually, emotionally and physically, in order to beat it. It is not unlike a war in that many, many innocent people suffer because of the selfishness and shortsightedness of others and in that it will take a coordinated and committed effort on the part of all of us to stop it.

In the meantime, you don't deserve it and you shouldn't lie back and accept it. You should fight. And one way to do that is being presented to you in your dreams.

In the dreams you've described, you are always the

victim, or the potential victim. You can take some of these images that your subconscious mind is presenting to you and use them as positive visualizations. The mind is a very powerful part of your being and here is an opportunity to put it to work. Try this: When you wake from one of your nightmares, immediately and consciously visualize an ending to the dream which shows you overcoming the victimizing situation you were in. For example, remember the dream in which you picked up a hitchhiker who had a gun and was trying to kill you? Well, upon waking you could have visualized that you stopped the car, grabbed the gun, and pushed the hitchhiker out of the car and then drove away without him.

I'm sure using a technique like this will defuse the anxiety you are feeling about these dreams and there is the possibility that successfully using this technique can improve your physical condition, as well. Lots of studies with cancer patients show really remarkable results when they use visualizations like the one I have described. Maybe your subconscious is "asking" you to try it.

And finally, as we discussed on the phone, my experience (which was as full of experimentation and limit-pushing as yours) ultimately led me to this conclusion: Only "material" problems are solved by material answers. Spiritual problems require spiritual answers. Your fear and anxiety may be distracted by sex, drugs, and rock n' roll, but they will not be relieved by the "things" of this world. The healing you need will be found only in your relationship with God. And only you can find that. The best way is by quietly asking for God's help.

I'm not recommending any particular path for you. I'm just saying, "Don't be afraid." As an interesting coincidence, today, Chris, my boss, received a brochure *of retreats from the Buddhist Shasta Abbey. Chris has always loved you and has been very good to you; I'm sure that he'd want you to have it. Chris goes there once a year and loves it. You may like it, too, except the Buddhists are a lot more finicky about smoking and coffee drinking than the Jesuits are. I know you enjoyed the Jesuit retreat you went to two years ago, and I'm sure you'd enjoy the Buddhist one, as well. The Buddhists retreats are cheaper, too.*

I love you a lot, Jonathan. You are much more incredibly brave and wonderful than you think you are. How could you deserve anything bad, when you've never deliberately hurt anyone. That something is a risk associated with a particular lifestyle does not mean it is "earned" when you get it. I forgive you everything, please forgive yourself.

Nick called his mom after he read the letter. "We got the letter you sent," he said. "Kim and I both read it over and over and we think it is the best letter you've written. And I'm going to go to the Buddhist retreat."

Aside from the lack of a cure, one of the many frustrations that PWAs and their families have dealt with over the years is the slow process for approval of new drugs by the Food and Drug Administration (FDA). Many have skirted the FDA by purchasing experimental drugs through buyers' clubs, organizations that obtain drugs in Mexico and Europe where approval processes are not as complicated as in the United States. Today, the approval process isn't nearly as lengthy as it has been in the past, and this is in part due to an organization called "Act Up." Act Up members, many of them HIV-positive, have marched, picketed, rallied, and interrupted government meetings to illustrate their frustration with government bureaucracy and their need and willingness to obtain experimental drugs immediately.

CHAPTER SEVEN

Medicine Games and Other Dilemmas

It was three weeks before Christmas and even the California air was turning nippy. Nick went to spend the night with his parents. He felt good, but had little energy. His mom turned out the sofa bed for him and he went to sleep. Half an hour or so later, he called out, "Mom, can you come here a minute?"

She put on her robe and went out to the living room. "What's the matter?"

"My feet are killing me." He grimaced as he spoke. "Could you rub them for me? Kim always rubs them for me at night and it really helps."

Luellen sat down and began to rub.

"You can rub pretty hard," he said.

Nick felt her thumbs push up and down the center of the soles of his feet. "Does that help?" she asked.

"A little," he said. But after a few more minutes he said, "You can stop now. They feel better. You don't rub feet as well as Kim does, but that helped."

He spent much of the next day playing Christmas carols on the piano and imitating Bing Crosby singing "White

Christmas." Kim came by and she, Nick, and Elizabeth decorated the tree. Nick talked his mom out of some decorations, and he and Kim went home to decorate a tree of their own.

Nick had stopped taking his medications before he went back East so he'd feel good enough to enjoy the trip. When he returned, he started taking them again, and as soon as he did, he became very sick. He couldn't keep food down, had a lot of intestinal pain, and was very weak. He had been back and forth to the hospital for all kinds of tests during Thanksgiving week. The doctor took him off all medications except dapsone and the MAI prophylaxis and put him on a lactose-free diet. Within a few days, the horrible symptoms disappeared. Nick never found out what caused them, but this much became clear: Nick could not take AZT anymore.

AZT is one of two antiviral drugs that had been approved for use by the Food and Drug Administration (FDA) at that time. The other was DDI. Antivirals slow or even reverse the spread of the HIV disease throughout the body and therefore prolong and enhance the quality of life. But they have serious side effects. Because a virus attaches itself to a cell so efficiently, the only way to kill a virus is to kill the host cell as well. The theory is if all the cells with virus are killed, the body will produce new cells without virus and the person will get better.

The theory works in well people, which is why early diagnosis is so important, but in sick people, the drug can't kill enough cells and the body can't reproduce new ones fast enough without huge doses being administered. AZT is not a smart drug. It can't discriminate between a healthy cell and an infected cell, so it kills good and bad cells alike. Human beings are made of cells; if enough cells die, the person dies. Taking AZT or any of the other antiviral drugs is tantamount to taking poison.

The side effects of DDI are different, and many people can take this drug longer with less damage, but the main side effect of DDI is neuropathy. If Nick took DDI, his neuropathy could have become so bad he might have ended up in a wheelchair.

There were two other drugs in the trial stage, then. One was another antiviral called DDC, similar to DDI, but which in many cases does not cause existing neuropathy to worsen. Nick's doctor had instructed him to begin taking DDC as soon as possible. Because the FDA had not yet approved this drug, a doctor could not write a prescription for it. Nick had to go through a buyers' club to buy it, and pay for it himself. Buyers' clubs are illegal. They must get their drugs in Europe and Mexico, and they cannot guarantee a regular supply. The cost for the drug was about thirty dollars for a one-week supply. It was expected that DDC would be approved within six months, but if Nick didn't get it then, he might not have been around to need it in six months.

The other drug was peptide T. Originally developed as an antiviral in 1986, its early trial results were not very dramatic, and it was all but forgotten except that many people who were suffering from neuropathy experienced a complete or nearly complete cessation of neurological symptoms while on the drug. This drug had no side effects and when used in conjunction with another antiviral, it seemed to increase the efficacy of the first antiviral, making the combined effects of the two drugs more powerful. If Nick could take DDC and peptide T, his neuropathy pain might go away and he might enjoy better quality and longer quantity of life. The buyers' club carried peptide T, but it cost two hundred dollars for a one-month supply.

Nick decided to buy the DDC from the buyers' club and wait for the peptide T.

On December 23, Kim and Nick went to his parents' house. The DDC had arrived a few days before, and he was taking one pill in the morning and one pill each night. He experienced no side effects and could not detect any increase in or worsening of his neuropathy. He believed the DDC would work. His attitudes about various therapies had always been neutral or negative. The fact that he believed something would work for him surely increased the chance that it would.

Toward the end of January, Nick's mom went up to Pacifica to visit with him. When she arrived, he was up and just beginning to clean the house.

Pacifica is a bedroom community about ten miles or so outside of San Francisco, situated on the cliffs overlooking the Pacific Ocean, just below the mouth of the bay. Nick and Kim rented a little bungalow atop a hill in an older neighborhood. Nick bragged that their house afforded a view of the sea to anyone game enough to climb up to the roof.

"Boy, it looks like you've been doing a lot of work here," Luellen said as she came into the house and surveyed the piles of books and clothes, bags of trash and cleaning supplies strewn about.

"Yeah," said Nick, "I've decided to clean up and make the place look nice." Nick and Luellen worked for several hours cleaning and organizing, rearranging furniture, and putting things away. Nick enjoyed having something other than AIDS to talk about — things like "What does Kim do with this?" and "Should I throw that away?"

In February, Nick got another bad report from the doctor. His CD4 count had dropped to 17. This time he took the news stoically. His weight was holding steady at 156 and his hair and skin looked healthy, but he was tired a lot. His blood sugar was low, he was growing a strange fungus in his mouth and, of course, the neuropathy was ever present.

Nick decided to try peptide T, and Kim bought him a two-week supply, which he began taking. He did not notice any improvement in this neuropathy, but he kept taking it anyway.

As he had planned, in February Nick went to the retreat at Shasta Abbey, a Buddhist monastery in the Cascade Mountains in northern California. He was very eager to tell his mom all about his experience when he got back. Everyone at the retreat, he told her, ate vegetarian meals in a very ritualized process that involved passing around bowls of strange grains and unusual vegetables. Nick said before everyone was served, all the food was cold. "But by the time it was okay to eat," he said, "everyone was so hungry, they didn't care whether the food was cold or what it tasted like. Which was a good thing," he said, laughing, "because none of it was that good.

"Everyone at the monastery has chores to do, too," he continued. "I told the monks I was sick, so they assigned me the job of sweeping a sidewalk. I'd start at one end, and by the time I got to the other end, the place where I started was covered with leaves again.

"I told the monk in charge of the grounds that it was impossible to keep the sidewalk clean, but he just smiled and said I was supposed to sweep the sidewalk, not keep it clean. So, I just swept it over and over until chore time was over. It was good to concentrate on doing something without having to worry about the results. I can't explain it, Mom, but just sweeping that sidewalk gave me such a feeling of peace."

The next week, Nick's urine turned brown, a symptom of hepatitis. He was panicky about this development and considered checking himself into a hospital for IV treatments of AZT, a drastic, end-stage measure. He had a liver-function test and another CD4 count. Luellen asked him to wait for the results before going into the hospital and he agreed.

The day after he had the tests, he invited his mom to come up and see him. Nick was in good shape that day. His weight and appetite were good, and his hair and skin looked healthy.

But he had very little energy and his neuropathy was much worse. In fact, he was hobbling rather than walking. He had been on peptide T for about ten days, but it hadn't helped. In spite of the difficulty he was having walking, he was determined to go shopping to get Kim a Valentine's Day gift. He finagled his mom into taking him to a mall near his home.

On the way to the mall he told her the one thing he would like to do in life was to get a college degree. "The only problem is," he said, "I think it would take me about six years to get one." He looked at her with searching eyes. "Do you think I have six years?"

"Of course you do," she said. Nick knew she was lying.

They went to a card shop that had a computer that allows one to print his own message on the card of his choice. Nick thought this terribly clever and spent an awfully long time getting the message to Kim just right. He also got her a heart covered box of Mrs. Field's cookies. He was getting tired and his feet were bothering him, so they decided to leave. But on the way out, they walked past a piano store, and nothing would do but that they go in and "price" pianos.

Nick wasn't dressed for shopping for $15,000 items, but he strode into the store undaunted and asked to see a sales person. His appearance was unimpressive, and he got the cold shoulder from the staff. After all, he hadn't brushed his hair in a few days, and under his olive-drab canvas coat that sometimes doubled as a bathrobe, he had on a dirty, frayed T-shirt. He was wearing mint-green sweatpants that had been cut off at the knee and out of which came skinny, little knobby legs that disappeared into huge, worn-out hiking boots.

He waited around for a salesperson a while, then sat down at the handsomest instrument in the establishment and began to play a most beautiful and ethereal song, an original of his. Everyone in the store stopped to listen and then the store manager herself came out to wait on Nick.

It was dark when Luellen dropped Nick off at his house.

As she left, she said, "Be sure to call me right away with the good news."

"What good news?" he asked.

"Your test results."

"You're going to be very disappointed," Nick said, "if it's bad news."

"It'll be good news," she said as she walked out the door. Nick smiled at her optimism.

The next day he called his mom from a pay phone at the clinic. "I have the best news of my life! I have forty-two CD4 cells!" After being on DDC for six weeks, and on DDC and peptide T in combination for ten days, his CD4 cells had more than doubled. His doctor was amazed. Nick was thrilled. He got his liver function results and his liver was fine. He did not have hepatitis. It had been one of the medications that had made his urine turn brown.

But AIDS is an up-and-down roller coaster. After four days of total elation over the jump in Nick's CD4 cells from seventeen to forty-two, and relief and gratitude over the fact that he did not have hepatitis, Nick developed terrible headaches and a black spot in the lower periphery of his vision. He went to the eye doctor the next day and found he had HIV retinopathy. There was no treatment for it.

In a few days, the headaches began to subside, and he got used to the black spot so that he hardly even noticed it. Nick was faithfully taking vitamins, and his meds and was feeling better everyday. The peptide T hadn't helped his neuropathy, but he continued to take it because he felt it was partly responsible for the jump in the CD4 cells the month before. Peptide T attaches itself to the same receptor on the CD4 cells to which the HIV virus attaches itself. If peptide T is there first, the virus can't attach itself and so the cell is protected.

As Nick became more interested in his recovery, he began to become more interested in doing things and in making plans. He and Kim began to plan a trip to Europe that summer.

Sitting around the coffee table at his mom's house one day, Nick spread out a map of Europe. He had a red marker and was making dots all over the map. "I want to go here," he'd say and make a dot. "And I want to go here." He would make another dot. "And here, and here, and there," Dot, dot, dot. With each dot, Kim's face became more stricken with a "how-are-we-going-to-pay-for-all-this" look. Nick caught a glimpse of Kim's face and without skipping a beat, put down the pen and folded up the map. "Actually," he said, "I want to go exactly where you want to go, Kimbo."

In the spring, Nick and Kim had moved out of their little house in Pacifica and into her father's house in Palo Alto. Nick started going to a support group. One of the guys in the group picked him up and took him to the meetings when Kim couldn't go. Nick was glad to have the chance to talk about AIDS with others who were going through it, too.

He was still waiting for FDA approval of DDC. But at the midnight hour, just before approval was to have occurred, the FDA recanted its approval, raided all the buyers' clubs, and confiscated all of the DDC so that none of it was available anywhere. Nick had only enough DDC to last through the end of March. The FDA ordered Hoffman LaRouche, the manufacturers of DDC, to do 5,000 more case studies before they would reconsider approval. Hoffman LaRouche set up more studies, but in the meantime they made the drug available on a compassionate-use basis to those who had been obtaining the drug through the buyers' clubs. Nick's doctor arranged for him to be a part of the compassionate-use program, so he was able to get DDC without paying for it.

Not long after, Nick and Kim invited his parents for dinner at the house in Palo Alto. After dinner, they sat in the living room talking for a while.

"Mom, Dad," said Nick, "I have a video that I want you guys to see."

They hesitated as it was getting late. "This movie is very

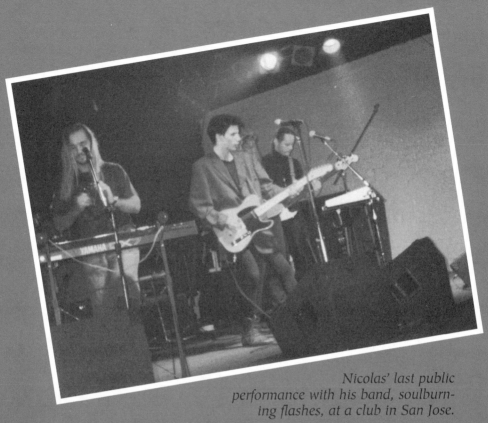

Nicolas' last public performance with his band, soulburning flashes, at a club in San Jose.

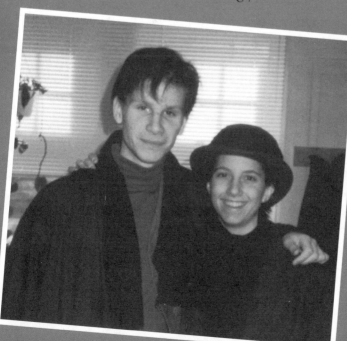

Nicolas and Kim at his Aunt Ellen's house in Philadelphia.

important to me," Nick insisted. "I've watched it about four times and I really need you guys to see it."

"Okay," they said.

The movie was *Jacob's Ladder,* a very difficult and brooding story of a Vietnam veteran in New York who is having hallucinations. The story was like a nightmare, and only at the end was the viewer sure that the theme of the movie was death. After the viewing, Nick was intent on knowing what his parents thought about the film. He was disappointed that they did not seem to be able to grasp its meaning or respond to his feelings. Nick thought the story to be an exposition of life after death, but he was unable to articulate that clearly to his parents. He had hoped the movie would act as a catalyst to a discussion of the topic of death, but his parents were uneasy and went home.

His disappointment was allayed when, a few days later, he received a letter from his mother:

We found Jacob's Ladder to be a very interesting film. I can see why you were moved and touched by this film and insisted that Dad and I watch it. Although, to be honest, if it hadn't been that you were so insistent that we see it, I don't think we would have watched it. But, we were glad you asked us to see it with you.

The point of the movie was not lost on us. We felt you were trying to tell us something about your coming to grips with death, the theme of the movie. I am of two minds about your interest in the film. Part of me is angry, because my twenty-two year old son is having to grapple with death and dying.

The other part of me is so very proud of you, Jonathan. The emotional and spiritual growth that you have shown in the past six months or so is simply astonishing. You are an amazing young man and my heart is full with love and pride.

She went on to talk about how in life human beings are separated from God and that death is a return to him.

I offer this to you as food for thought. If you consider death as a return to the Unity, Eternity, and Love from which we came, then the fear simply is inconsistent. We are not going to a final judgment by a jealous god, we are returning to the loving Creator who created us and loves us as we are. Our journey here is simply to prepare for that return.

Nick appreciated her letter. He was relieved that he had communicated some of what he was feeling through the movie and was glad his parents got it.

ost PWAs understandably experience periods of denial and anger. By finding some positive way to channel their energies, however, many find that their health issues stabilize. They renew their interests in the world outside of their disease and rediscover their ability to enjoy living. For some, such as Nick, this positive energy comes from educating others about AIDS. For others, it may be through art or writing or political activism. The next time you think about your local AIDS agency, understand that it provides more than information. It provides life!

Anger

As the guilt began to subside, anger took hold. Nick was no stranger to anger, having spent most of his teen years being angry at his parents, teachers, and the world for their real and imagined failings. Now he had a more tangible and vicious enemy — the virus which was sucking his life away.

He struggled to deal with his anger in many ways. Some of his struggle was reflected in the music he was writing.

Land of the Free

by Nicolas J. Trevor

> *i hear the glass break through*
> *it's the world outside*
> *i can't believe you're not burning inside*
> *how can you live day to day*
> *without blowing up to a screaming rage?*
> *screaming a vengeance it's been too long*

without a blowout protest
look at our world
is there anyone inside?
is it beginning to hurt?
is there anyone in the land of the free?
i was brought up in a crossfire with a dirty face
and i get sick and i get tired of this american race
and your narrow minded malcontent
you still don't know why you can't look me in the eye
and tell me what went wrong
talk about democracy . . .
talk about money . . .
talk about aids . . .
people die do people love
and your bulldozer government
making up new problems
so we can fight without a cause,
go to bed and sleep well . . .

—From the soulburning flashes' album
Screaming Psychosis

His anger began to color every aspect of his life, including his relationship with Kim. One afternoon, he was lying on the couch at the house in Palo Alto, trying to sleep, when Kim came home. He heard her come in, but he was tired and didn't feel like acknowledging her. He was aware that she looked at him and then walked away. He didn't say anything. He was angry. He was angry because she was well and he was sick. She could go out and do what she pleased, while he lay in bed.

Kim went into the next room where their friend Paul was. Nick heard them start to talk in the casual way that friends talk about nothing. They sounded normal, as though they had not a care in the world, and Nick began to resent the happy sounds he heard coming from their direction. Soon he was enraged. He couldn't stand it anymore. He got up and went into the room where they were and started yelling at them.

In an uncharacteristic show of paranoia, he began to accuse Kim of having an affair with Paul. They argued, and then Kim told Nick to go home for a few days. She went to call his mother while Nick retreated to the bedroom.

The next day, Luellen went to Palo Alto to pick him up and found Nick too weak to get out of bed without help. He couldn't put on his shoes by himself, and it took both Paul and Luellen to carry him out to the car.

For the first twenty minutes of the trip home he was quiet. Then, he spoke, "Mom, what's wrong with me? Why do I feel this way?" Tears started to roll down his cheeks.

"Nick," she said, reaching across to wipe a tear away, "there are a few things going on with you. You're depressed. And you're entitled to your depression. But a big part of the problem is all the dilaudid you're taking."

"I know I'm taking too much," he said. "But I don't have anything else to do. All my friends go out to clubs and have a good time. Either I can't go, or I go and don't feel well and have to come home early."

Dilaudid is a powerful narcotic, a kind of synthetic heroin that his doctor had prescribed for pain. Nick was taking the medication not only to dull the pain of his neuropathy but to dull the emotional pain and anger he was experiencing.

"The dilaudid is only making things worse; it is increasing your depression, not making it better," Luellen said. "And it makes you do and say things that are unkind. You're hurting Kim." She watched him as she drove along the freeway.

"I know, and I'm mad at myself about that."

"Well, don't be mad at yourself, just stop."

He was quiet for a while and then he began to sob. "Mom, what's happening to me? I'm so scared."

She squeezed his leg. "You're developing a drug dependency again," she said, matter-of-factly. "I know you need to take it for the pain, but you must try to not take so much."

That night, his mother read to him from <u>The Color of Light</u> (an AIDS meditation book) until he fell asleep. The next day, he awoke determined not to overdo the pain medication anymore. His depression lifted, but the root of it, his anger, was still there.

Two days after his mom had picked him up, Nick spoke at Gilroy High School. The high school had asked ARIS, a non-profit agency that provided support and services to people with AIDS and HIV, to send a speaker to address their family issues committee. Aris asked Nick to go. He was nervous; he had gone to Gilroy High and he expected he might see people he knew. He wasn't sure how he would handle that.

The first person he met was the school nurse. "I remember you," she said to Nick. "You stole a pack of cigarettes from Longs Drug Store, and the police caught you and brought you back to school. You told everyone you were sick and you spent the whole day in my office."

He recognized a lady whose daughter he had dated in high school. By the time the room was full, there were a lot of people there whom he knew.

Nick took a seat on a folding chair in the middle of the room and crossed his slender legs nonchalantly. Clearly he enjoyed these presentations, and whatever trepidations he may have had about "going home" dissipated.

He began telling his story. By the middle of his second sentence, the group was spellbound, completely enthralled by Nick and what he had to say.

"When I was younger," he told them, "I was just like all teenagers. I thought I could do whatever I wanted and nothing bad would ever happen to me. I knew about AIDS, but I didn't think it would happen to me. It was the kind of thing that happened to other people.

"So, I didn't take care of myself. I didn't have safe sex. I shared needles. I was having fun. I just didn't think about what could happen."

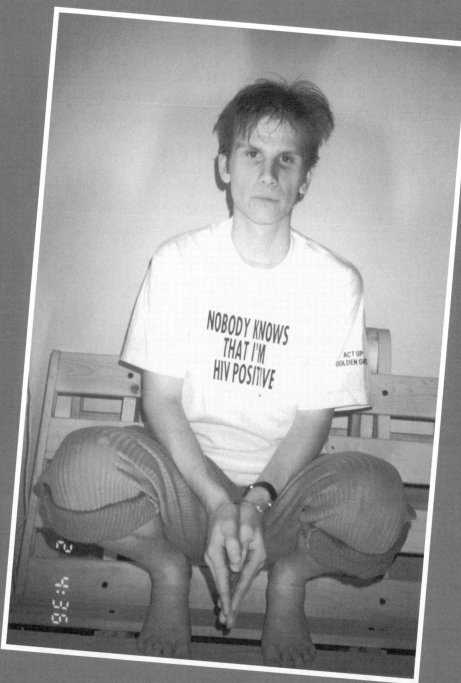

Nicolas at home in Pacifica.

He finished his story. Then he began to give some specifics about the disease.

"Basically, there are very few ways to become infected with HIV. The most 'popular' way is by having unprotected sex with someone who is infected. The chances of being infected by female-to-male transmission are about 1 in 500 and one in two hundred for male-to-male or male-to-female transmission. But don't let those numbers lull you into thinking you can go out and have sex 199 times and be safe. It's like the lottery." Nick smiled. "Somebody always wins.

"Sharing needles with an infected person is another way. Health care providers can be at risk if they have an open cut that is exposed to infected blood products. And infected mothers can pass the virus to their children while they are pregnant, during delivery, and by breast-feeding. But those are the only ways to become infected. You can't get AIDS by kissing someone with AIDS, or drinking out of a glass they've used, or anything like that.

"What you need to remember," he concluded, "is that there are only four vehicles of transmission: sperm, blood and blood products, vaginal secretions, and mother's milk."

Then he opened up the discussion for questions. The group of parents, teachers, and a few students asked him about everything, and he answered each question with poise and dignity.

One of the students and a teacher started to argue about handing out condoms at school. Nick broke in and said, "This isn't about morality; this is about safety. You don't have to pass out condoms, and you don't have to encourage kids to have sex. But you must let them know that if they decide to have sex there are ways to do it safely. And you have to let them know where to get condoms. When I was in high school, everybody knew which gas station rest rooms had condoms, but they didn't want to go to those places to get them. Let kids know that they can get condoms at any AIDS services agency."

After the presentation, the people came up to shake his hand or hug him, and the woman whose daughter had dated Nick shook his hand.

"That felt real good," Nick said to his mom as they walked back to the car after the presentation was over. Nick had been wallowing in self-pity and anger for some weeks, but giving his talk made him feel something he hadn't felt in a long time: worthwhile. It was valuable to help others. It invigorated him and it made the depression and the anger go away. The anger would continue to ebb and swell, but now he had a weapon to fight it. Now he didn't have to be a victim of his own pain.

He began to get involved in his recovery again and he cut down on the pain medication. He started taking the rest of his meds correctly and taking all his vitamins, although he gave up completely on the peptide T. His doctor referred him to the pain clinic at Stanford in the hope that they would be able to find a treatment that would offer him some relief from the pain in his feet. And he began to make himself available for more presentations about AIDS/HIV for young people.

From the outset, AIDS was not a popular disease. It didn't attract spokespeople and wasn't the recipient of well-organized telethons. Indeed, in the beginning it was largely ignored and treated as a "gay disease." Because gays were already marginalized and despised, it was easy for the mainstream population to dismiss the disease. There are those who say that if it had struck the heterosexual population with the same vengeance that it struck the homosexual population, money to combat it would have been immediately forthcoming. But in Western Europe and America the virus typically did not attack heterosexuals; its first targets were homosexuals.

We will never know if immediate action might have stemmed the AIDS epidemic. What we do know is that those who acquired it were stigmatized. AIDS and the verbal blame from religious conservatives gave homophobic people an excuse to express their fears (Gilbert Herdt and Andrew Boxer, *Children of Horizons*, (Boston: Beacon Press, 1993), p. 60), and they did so by beating up those perceived to be gay, by burning down the homes of PWAs, by ostracizing not just PWAs but their entire families as well. Whether people were gay or not, once diagnosed with HIV or AIDS, they "became" part of the gay community.

CHAPTER NINE

On Dealing with Sexuality

As a young man living with AIDS, Nick also had to live with people's biases and prejudices about not only the disease itself but also sexuality. Most people he met assumed he was either a hemophiliac or gay.

For Nick, the question of his sexuality, or sexual orientation (a term he hated), had long been an issue. He wasn't sure exactly when he began to notice that this was a question which had to be answered, but by the time he was fifteen, or so, it had become a major issue for him.

His angst over his sexual identity became evident when he was sixteen and in the psychiatric hospital. During one of the weekly family therapy meetings, the psychiatrist mentioned casually that Nick and his roommate had been found that morning sleeping on the floor together with their teddy bears. The conversation continued on for a while and then the doctor interrupted.

"Excuse me, Mrs. Reese," he said to Nick's mother, "I have to clarify something. A few minutes ago, I told you the nurse found Nick sleeping with another boy, and you never batted an eye. Don't you have a reaction to that statement?" Nick feigned disinterest but was paying close attention.

"Not really. Should I have a reaction?" asked Luellen.

Nick's behavior at the hospital had been outrageous. It was easy for Nick to assert his independence within the confines of a structured environment. He could convince himself that he was free simply by breaking all the rules. Sleeping on the floor with his teddy bear and his roommate had just been part of the game. Nick wondered if his mother knew that.

"I think most parents would have a reaction to that kind of information," said the doctor. "Some would even have a violent reaction. The implication here is that Nick might be a homosexual."

"Were they having sex?" Luellen asked, looking the doctor squarely in the face.

Nick glanced back at the doctor, who now seemed a little unsettled. "No," said the doctor.

"Then why should I assume that Nick is homosexual?"

Nick could see his mom and his doctor had moved beyond therapy and were now engaged in a duel, which he found quite entertaining.

"You shouldn't, but how would you feel if he were?" said the psychiatrist. Nick shifted his body away from his mother. He was sure there were no limits to her love for him, but for just a moment he was afraid of what her answer might be.

"It wouldn't make any difference to me. He is still my son, and I would love him just the same," Luellen declared to the doctor. Her voice softened and she gazed at Nick. "I think Nick is in the process of discovering his sexuality and that's normal."

The psychiatrist was looking at her as though she had a rooster on her head. Nick was watching her out of the corner of his eye and smiling.

"It wouldn't bother you at all," said the psychiatrist.

"Look, Doctor," she said, "no parent wants their child to be a homosexual. In this world, all other things being equal, the life of a homosexual is a much more difficult row to hoe than the life of a heterosexual, given AIDS, homophobia, discrimination, and so on. But if my son is gay, he's gay, and I would love him just the same."

And that was the end of that conversation. He wouldn't say so, but Nick was proud of his mother for her response to the doctor.

While Nick was in the hospital, a complete psychological work up was done on him. He met with his doctor to go over the results. "It would seem," his doctor said, "that you are confused about your sexuality."

Nick nodded. His doctor continued talking as he perused the psychologist's report. "But it seems, also, that you have a strong belief that your ultimate happiness depends upon having a girlfriend. How do you feel about that?"

Nick thought it over for a minute. "I'm not sure," he said.

"Do you have lots of girlfriends?" the doctor asked.

"Yeah," Nick said. "I always have a girlfriend."

In high school, guys often make cruel jokes about other guys. Nick was one of the ones the others made jokes about. Though he always had a girlfriend, other boys were forever calling him a faggot and beating him up. He didn't know why he attracted this kind of attention. However, this barbaric treatment did cause him to withdraw and become very distrustful and disdainful of many of his fellow students. He developed a very small and tight group of friends who were for the most part social outcasts as he was. Some of his friends were gay, and he found that he felt very comfortable in the "gay world."

About a year into his fight with AIDS, Nick said to his mother that he thought he had decided, once and for all, that he was bisexual.

"How do you feel about that?" she asked him.

They were sitting in the backyard of his parents' home. Nick crossed his legs and wrapped his slender fingers around his knee. "Actually," he said, "I would rather be one or the other. Being bisexual seems neither here nor there to me, like I'm on the fence."

"So, pick one side or the other," she suggested.

"That's just it; I can't."

"Well, if you had to pick one over the other, which would it be?

He thought about it for a while and said, "I'm not sure, but if I could only be straight or gay, I think I would choose being gay."

"Why?"

"Well, for one thing," he said, laughing, "the best sex I've ever had was with men."

"That's not true," his mother said. "The best sex you ever had was with Mary Chavez."

A silly grin crossed his face as he remembered his girl-friend of four years past. "Yeah," he said "that was the best sex I ever had."

"Besides," his mother said, "I don't think that who you enjoy having sex with the most determines your sexuality; your sexuality determines who you enjoy having sex with."

"I don't follow you," Nick said.

Luellen told him about a gay friend of hers who told her that before he knew he was gay he could have sex with a woman and find it to be enjoyable, but when it was over he wanted to run. When he began to have sex with men, he wanted to cuddle up and stay all night. "So," she concluded, "I think that it is the kind of person that you want to cuddle up with, not the kind you want to have sex with, that is impor-tant. And in your case, although you have had physical rela-tionships with men, you only select women as significant oth-ers. You only cuddle up and stay all night with girls."

"So, you're saying I'm straight," he said.

"I think so," his mother said.

"Maybe you just want me to be straight."

"Maybe. But answer this: who do you want to spend the rest of your life with?"

"Kim," he said without hesitation.

"Well, in that case, wouldn't it be more convenient if you were straight?"

Nick smiled at his mother's logic, but her arguments did not settle the issue for him. What was true for him was that Kim was the one for him and had his illness not so infringed on their life together in so many horrible and insidious ways, he would have loved her and cherished her for many years. But that didn't mean he was straight as far as he was concerned.

"You know," his mother said, "just because AIDS and homosexuality go hand-in-hand in the minds of most people, when people find out you have AIDS, they ask me if you are gay."

"What do you say?"

"Well, I used to say, 'No, he isn't gay.' But now I tell them it's none of their business."

One day, Nick's extended family was gathered at his mom's house for a barbecue, and, as was their wont to do, they sat around the dining room table settling all the great problems of the world. The conversation turned to homosexuality. Nick, of course, led the pro side of the discussion.

Karin, his evangelical aunt, spoke up, "Well, in the Bible, it says . . ."

Nick wanted to hear what Karin had to say, but his mother interrupted. "You can't really go by the Bible. After all, in the whole book, there are only seven references to homosexuality, four in the Old Testament and three in the letters of Saint Paul. We can forget the Old Testament," she said, "because taking those references in the context of the time and culture in which they were written, understanding what relevance they have to here and now is beyond us. As to Saint Paul, he lumps homosexuality with a variety of other sexual activities which he condemns, not so much for their supposed perversion, but for the distraction they cause in keeping people from readying themselves for the Second Coming, which Paul was expecting momentarily. Paul was dissuading his followers from sex altogether, as being unnecessary, in view of the imminent end of time."

Nick had never heard this point of view and was very interested by what his mother had to say.

"But," she continued, "God does speak to us in other ways, and the better argument against homosexuality would be found in nature. Homosexuality does not exist in nature and therefore would not seem to be a creation of God."

"Mom, how can you say that? You don't think God created homosexuals?" Nick said.

"No, I'm not saying that," she said. "I'm just saying I don't think he created homosexuality because it doesn't exist in nature."

Before Nick could retaliate, his Aunt Janet's boyfriend, a biologist, entered the conversation. "Actually, you are not entirely correct," he said to Luellen. "Most species do not practice homosexuality, but there are a couple species of primates that do."

This was news to everyone at the table. Then the biologist added, "In fact, it seems that these primates practice homosexuality as a response to their habitat being over populated."

No one had a response to this information, and the conversation turned to other matters.

A few weeks later, Nick heard about Simon LeVey's study, in which LeVey had discovered biological differences between the hypothalamus glands of gay men and straight men. Nick was incensed by the ramifications of this limited and controversial study. "If sexuality were proven to be biological in origin," he told his mother, "extremists would be tempted toward 'cures' and 'prevention.' Babies with 'gay hypothalamus glands' might even be aborted." Nick was pleased to see that his mom was as horrified by this prospect as he was. "LeVey's study was very small and actually proves nothing," he said.

His mother looked at him thoughtfully. "Actually, it causes the whole issue to fall neatly in place for me," she said. "I can honestly say that I never chose to be heterosexual. I was born this way. If I were born heterosexual, then perhaps sexual orientation is biological. If so, it must come from God. If it exists in nature, as Janet's boyfriend says, then it must be natural and part of the purpose of man."

"What difference does it make why people are gay," said Nick. "Some people just are, and they shouldn't be discriminated against because of it."

"I never said people should be discriminated against because they are gay," his mother said. "But you must recognize that for many people, sexuality is a moral issue."

"Well, it shouldn't be," said Nick.

Nick never did determine if he was gay, straight, or bi. In the final analysis, he decided that it just didn't matter.

Those of us who are healthy usually take our daily routines for granted. We get up in the morning, exercise, go to school, run errands, and meet with friends. Only when we are robbed of our routines do we appreciate them. The ordinariness of day-to-day activities is extraordinary to a person with an illness. A person with AIDS marks time with medical appointments, their supply of AZT, and the last hospitalization. Most hope for a little normalcy in their lives, to know that Monday morning is British Literature or that Wednesday afternoon is bowling with buddies. When they feeling well and can experience life's ordinary routines, they are almost able to push aside the reality of AIDS — at least for a time.

CHAPTER TEN

A Touch of Normalcy

In the summer of 1992, Nick began to feel better and he became more active. That summer he took a literature class at Foothill College. He became a member of the board of directors for the ARIS Project; he was already on their speaker bureau. He began giving more presentations on AIDS at high schools.

July 19 was the eighth annual San Francisco AIDS Walk. Nick's dad marched in the AIDS Walk carrying a sign that read, on one side, "While Mr. Bush is fishing . . ." The other side read, "I'm walking for my son's life." The sign, of course, referred to the president's trip to Montana that week, and the administration's apparent lack of interest in AIDS research and funding.

Nick had been at a retreat for people with AIDS that weekend. He knew his dad was planning to walk, but he didn't know about the sign. When he got home late Sunday night, he flipped on the news and quite by chance, he hit channel 4. There was his dad.

At 10:06 P.M., Nick called his parents. "I saw my dad!" he

said excitedly. "He was carrying a sign. It said 'I'm walking for my son's life.'"

"That's right," his mother said. "He walked for you."

"I was just calling to tell Dad thank you, and to tell him that I love him."

Nick knew he was a lucky guy, even if he did have AIDS. He was lucky because he had friends and family who loved him, and he was lucky because he had Kim. Many nineteen-year-old girls might have left a guy who was diagnosed with AIDS, but Nick knew that Kim did not desert her friends and she was not going to desert him. Every moment that she was able, she was with him. And when he went home to his parents' house, every moment she wasn't at work or at school, she was there with him. He loved her so much. He loved to open his eyes after a nap and see her curled up on a chair with a book open on her lap. She made this nightmare almost bearable for him.

He and Kim finally left her father's home in Palo Alto and found a place of their own in Santa Cruz. In August they moved in and shortly thereafter started at their respective colleges.

Nick didn't have a phone right away, so he wrote to his mother.

August 25, 1992

Dear Mom,

I'm currently undergoing a sort of giddy, almost childlike, excitement. Right now, I am very happy.

I know I've felt like this before, but it has been a long time and I can't seem to remember any particular incidences that were nearly like what I'm experiencing now. I'll try to explain, but forgive me if I run on or sound jumbled.

So . . . I'm just tickled pink at the fact that 10(9+2)

= 10 x 9 + 10 x 2 and that I know why. I also know that the difference between the two halves of that equation is the distribution property. I feel proud of knowing this. It's nearly indescribable. I did last night's algebra homework last night, then today, I spent an hour doing it again in the math tutorial lab. I got it right both times. I'm understanding this shit.

I feel strongly that if I put in some extra hours in the math lab, regularly, there will be no question that I will get an "A" in math. But only if I put in extra hours with a tutor. This type of mathematics DOES NOT come naturally to me (as do so many other things).

This will take work, but I've figured that out, too. But more about that later. In the meantime . . .

I am ecstatic about the fact that I know who begot Zeus, why and how and what significance that has in all of Western culture. I can also tell you that St. Augustine used Platonic ideology as the method for his theory of "universality" which in Latin is "catholic." The fact that Augustine gave the Church something to do, came directly from Plato. And it stayed that way until Thomas Aquinas came along. Now Thomas, like Augustine, was very much into Plato, but that was nothing compared to his love of Aristotle, especially Nichodemacean ethics. The Church accepted this theory of Thomas' and the Church has been the same ever since.

Funny that during the Inquisition anyone found worshipping Apollo or Dionysus would have been burned at the stake when the men that had laid the groundwork for Catholic theology praised Apollo and Dionysus.

But, that's nothing compared to what Freud did with the Greeks. But enough said about that. Summary: I really enjoy the topic of Classical Greece.

Now, for the whammy — I've gone three days without a cigarette! and as a testament to that, I've enrolled in a fitness and exercise class. A little running and jumping will do me some good. I actually attend this class for the first time tomorrow (8/26). >Which reminds me, wish Liz a very happy b-day.<

Altogether, I think P.E. is a good idea.

I've got a full load this time, no fluff — all my classes are G.E. required with lots of work. Now, as I said before, I have figured this out. In all of my scholastic life — none of the idea of really knowing how to succeed in school ever made sense to me, until now. The key, I'm finding, is immersion. Nothing else. My whole existence must be school. The situation I am in caters to just that.

The reason I never did this before was alternative prioritization (and naiveté). The past was filled with tumultuous changes in the way I identified my whole existence; i.e., I was a pimply outcast, therefore school sucked. My drunk father didn't care about my school-work but rather looked at school as free daycare, therefore school sucked. I was busy being rebellious, therefore school sucked. I wanted to get laid, therefore school sucked. I was an egotist who knew more than anyone else, therefore school sucked. There are thousands of things, yet none of them got me very far.

I now find that if I identify myself as a student, then school becomes easily doable. As I completely immerse myself, I can do nothing but succeed. That's always been the case with me, whether it was being the outcast, or the rebel, or the artist, or the addict. It has always been all or nothing. Maybe you'd call that compulsion, but in art and ascetics we learn that compulsions aren't in and of themselves bad. Compulsive people have com-posed symphonies, created masterful works of art, built bridges and been good students. Do straight-A students look obsessive-compulsive? Damn near always.

So, as long as I'm all the way into what I'm doing,

I'll make it. I wake up, have coffee, go to school, study, sleep and, so far, I'm enjoying it. I'm limiting as much extraneous distraction as possible.

Mark my words: "I intend to make honor roll this year."

So, I need to put forth a question to you: How much of a role do you want to take in my education? This is a multipoint question that I can explain to you later, but for now, let me just say that it has a great deal to do with U.C.S.C.[University of California at Santa Cruz]. U.C.S.C. is becoming much more of a reality. This is both exciting and scary, but it is also the content of my next letter.

In the meantime, I'm very happy and I'm feeling good. Yes, I feel good, and yes, I am taking all of my vitamins, and eating as well as I can.

Things are good.
I love you
your son

P.S. I was inspired to write on account of we still have no phone.

The last weekend in August, his parents went to see Nick and Kim in their new little home in Santa Cruz. It was a small, funky little cottage, very "Nick and Kim."

When they arrived, his parents found Nick sitting on the front steps drinking a cup of coffee and smoking a cigarette. "This," he announced, "is my last cigarette, so let me enjoy it." Nick never smoked again.

They were still in the process of getting settled, and Nick was feeling good. He was full of "decorating plans" and Kim was planning a garden. They gave Bill and Luellen the grand tour and the four of them visited for the afternoon.

That evening, Kim went out for a while. As he was chatting with his parents and sorting through unpacked boxes, Nick bemoaned, in a light-hearted way, the great chasm between his disregard for material possessions and Kim's attachment to hers. Nick was utilitarian and only owned things which he used and used all the things he owned. Kim, on the other hand, was a collector. Going through one of the unpacked boxes, he pulled out a gadget meant to be fastened to a door so that one might hang clothes on it. "This," he said, "is quintessential Kim." He laughed the laughter of someone without a care in the world.

"One day," he continued, "when we were living in Saratoga, she decided to get organized, so she bought this. We took it with us when we moved to Pacifica. We took it when we moved to Palo Alto. And we brought it here." He waved the apparatus in the air. "It's still in the package. She's never used it, but it goes with us wherever we go." He grinned broadly as he dropped it into a box and said, "Quintessential Kim."

He started at Cabrillo College, taking philosophy, English, library science, math, and adaptive physical education, which is P.E. for handicapped people. Nick loved his P.E. class. All of the people in it were much more physically limited than he. Most of them were in wheelchairs and many of them were developmentally disabled as well. Many in the class thought Nick was one of the teacher's aides because he was in better shape than they. They were always asking him to help them on and off the machines. He enjoyed them and he enjoyed helping them.

Nick bought himself a new pair of fancy white sneakers to wear to class. One of the guys with Down's Syndrome was very enamored of Nick's new shoes and asked him where he got them.

"I got them at Kmart," Nick told him.

"What's Kmart?" asked the boy.

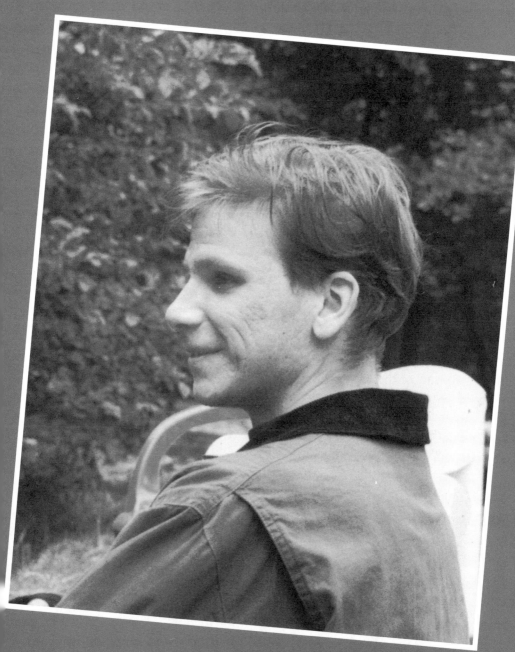

Nicolas, 22, in his favorite green coat on a camping trip in Big Sur.

"It's a store where you can buy things like shoes," Nick answered.

"Where is it?"

"It's on Forty-first Avenue," said Nick.

"How do you get there?"

"You take the bus."

A few days later, Nick was on one of the machines where you lift weights with your legs by hooking your feet under the weights. The boy with Down's watched him for a while and then said, "You are lifting a very heavy weight."

"Yes," said Nick, "I am."

Then with great awe in his voice, the other kid said, "It must be those shoes."

Elizabeth's best friend, Laurel, was in Nick's philosophy class. She told Liz that Nick was the smartest guy in the class. Laurel said she moved her seat closer to him so that his "smarts" would rub off on her.

One day, Nick was riding the bus home from school when Lauren, his fifteen-year-old cousin got on the bus. They rode part of the way home together. He was so impressed by how smart and grownup his cousin was. He reflected how odd it was that when you see your cousins at family gatherings, they're just cousins, but when you meet them out in the world, they're like real people.

August, September, and the early part of October were a glorious time because Nick felt well. He was enjoying life, school, his little house, and Kim. And he was also keeping busy giving presentations for young people about AIDS.

In mid-October, he was invited by the San Jose Diocesan AIDS Office to speak to the youth groups from various parishes in the diocese. He was part of a panel of young people that included an unwed teenage mother, a recovering drug addict, and others. He was the person with AIDS.

Nick spoke eloquently about his experience and the disease. After his talk, he opened up the discussion for questions from the audience. Most of the kids were supportive, but a few of them were uncomfortable. One boy got up and expressed extreme surprise at the fact that Nick had a girlfriend. (Nick had spoken of Kim.) The young man said, "I know this sounds awful, but if my girlfriend had AIDS, I'd drop her."

"You're honest, and that's good," said Nick. "But there would be no reason to drop a friend just because that friend had AIDS. I'm still me and Kim isn't going to let the fact that I'm sick come between us."

"Yeah," said the boy, "but AIDS is …"

"I know, it's scary," said Nick. "But we're careful. We don't do anything that endangers Kim. Look, people with AIDS are people. We have feelings just like everybody else, and the people who love us don't let the disease get in the way."

Everyone in the auditorium was quiet, then the boy spoke again. "I feel like I should give you a hug," he said. Nick started toward him, but the boy shook his head and sat down.

Nick shrugged. After the discussion was over, several of the kids came up to him and shook his hand and a few even hugged him. These kids didn't get what Nick was telling them. It is a tough message to give to kids, that they are vulnerable. When adults tell them, they don't believe it. When they saw the truth, embodied in Nick, as they did, they often couldn't confront it.

A few days later, Nick had another opportunity to share the truth with young people. He was invited to participate in a documentary for young people about young people with HIV.

He enjoyed being with others his own age who were HIV positive. (He was the only one in the group with full-blown AIDS.) He didn't think the documentary's producers were going to use much of him in the video, and he didn't think he had done very well. He would have to wait and see.

HIV and AIDS remain, in many ways, mysteries. The time between infection and AIDS-related illness or illnesses varies from person to person, and doctors don't know exactly why. But with new treatments, some people who test positive for HIV may show no signs of illness for eight to eleven years and more. They may look healthy, but inside the virus is ticking away. For others, the window of apparent health is only a few months. ("HIV Infection and AIDS: Are You at Risk?" (Centers for Disease Control and Prevention, U.S. Public Health Service, 1994), and the CDC AIDS Hotline, 1996)

Because the disease baffles science, many of the treatments are experimental, and it has been difficult for the average family practitioner to keep up with developments. For this reason, PWAs have had to educate themselves about opportunistic infections that are common threats, their various treatments, and potential side effects. And in many instances, a PWA will know more than the professional health-care giver.

CHAPTER ELEVEN

Dealing with the Illness

Medicine Man
by Nicolas J. Trevor

Look at us all.
Feel the moment
When it's 3 a.m.
And I'm soaked in sweat,
Like when I'm too sick to sleep
And I'm too tired to fight about it.
You call me crazy,
Then come along for the ride.
> *Say why — Ask why*
> *No way — don't take my life away*
> *One time — last time*
> *No way I'm gonna give it away.*

You look inside me,
Feel that I am dangerous.
You sound so silly

Saying I'm courageous.
Oh, come invade me.
I'm lying on my back
Like there's nothing in my heart
When the angels come and save me.
      Medicine Man
      Come to me in the morning
      With my feet on fire
      And my head so distorted.

AIDS is a terrible disease and a terrible epidemic. One of the things that makes it formidable is the fact that it seems invisible. Nobody knows anybody with AIDS or HIV, or so they think.

Before he was diagnosed, Nick knew no one with AIDS, not personally. After he and his family began to talk about their own situation to others, they found many people whose lives had been touched by this horrible disease. The younger brother of a friend of his dad's had died of AIDS; Sean, who ran a sandwich shop Nick used to frequent, died of AIDS; the nephew of a friend of his mom's had died of AIDS; the brother of a neighbor had AIDS; the daughter and son-in-law of a woman his mother worked with had AIDS; a dear family friend was HIV positive. Before Nick began telling these folks about his own illness, all these people had been silent about their own situations. Nick wondered how many people don't know they are acquainted with folks fighting this disease because people are afraid to talk.

In December, Nick's condition so worsened that he was admitted to the hospital in Santa Cruz. He was dehydrated, his nausea was so bad that he had not kept down a meal in days, and he was losing weight rapidly. He was jaundiced and itching all over from jaundice.

The physician treating him in the hospital was the only "AIDS doctor" in Santa Cruz, but he declined to treat Nick upon his release from the hospital because Nick was on Medi-Cal. Nick was beside himself. He took it personally that the Santa Cruz doctor wouldn't treat him. He was hurt deeply by this glitch in the medical system, and he was scared.

Nick was in the cancer ward, since the hospital had no AIDS ward. One of the nurses commented to him that he had an opportunistic infection. He wanted to know which one. The nurse didn't know what he was talking about when he started listing off the various options.

"Do I have CMV?" he demanded. "MAI? Toxoplasmosis? Cryptococcosis?"

The nurse hadn't heard of these diseases. "All I know," she said, "is when a person with cancer has a fever, it means they have an opportunistic infection. And it's the same with people who have what you have," said the nurse, who apparently couldn't say the word AIDS.

"No, it isn't," said Nick. "People with AIDS have fevers all the time. If I do have an opportunistic infection, I want to know which one I have."

The nurse scurried away and never came back. Nick called the Director of Patient Services at the hospital and offered to do an in-service training for the nursing staff about AIDS. His offer was declined. He was tested for CMV and MAI, but the tests came back negative.

He wrote a letter to his doctor in a desperate attempt to regain a modicum of control over his health care.

Nick's Idea For His Current Treatment

TO: Dr. Donald Polanski & Anybody else who cares
FROM: Nicolas Trevor

Dear Dr. Polanski,
I truly feel that I am now ready enough to be discharged as soon as possible, and to continue the infu-

sions of erythromycin in my home by a visiting nurse. I will also keep taking whatever you feel I should be on. Now, as far as my liver treatment goes I am perfectly able to make the drive up there as much as you need me to work with you and Geoff, and Dr. Farley and the other specialist you mentioned from UCSF. But if you or Farley need regular labs, I'd rather do them at the Met West in Santa Cruz. All this will take is one phone call to Santa Cruz Public Health Dept., and NOT San Mateo County's under-budgeted health care system.

First of all Santa Cruz has a much higher budget than San Mateo right now. They are much better about visiting nurses and supplying wheel chairs and so on. However, to stay legal and proper, you need to order all of the things that I need right now through Santa Cruz Public Health. The woman with whom you need to speak is Joan Skyler, she is very familiar my case.

I also need to know if rather than giving me four separate infusions a day, if it would be feasible to just have one long infusion a day instead of four infusions a day every six hours? Perhaps you could raise the dosage and just have one long infusion every day. Is this safe if I also continue the high doses of trimetheprin and dapsone. This would very comfortable for me, and the visiting nurse would only have to come to administer the infusion once a day. Again, all you would need to do is make a call to Joan Skyler and she'll take care of everything. Please tell me if this method will be as safe and effective as staying here at the hospital.

OK, now the particulars of what exactly I need from you now (and by the way, I don't want to come across as a selfish know-it-all, I just want to make my health care easier on both of us):

1. A visiting nurse once a day
2. One wheelchair

3. An OK to have my regular blood work done at Met West in Santa Cruz

4. An order for all the equipment that the nurse may need — i.e. infusion equipment, etc.

I feel that you should be able to do this all with just one phone call to Joan Skyler at the Santa Cruz Health Department. I truly believe that this route will make everybody happy, especially San Mateo County, myself, and you. Also, bear in mind that I am perfectly willing to make the trip up here so that you can see me regularly as well, we just need to work out a schedule of how often you want me to actually come in for an appointment.

Thank you so much for all that you've done for me. I'm trying hard now not to sound demanding, it's just that we can work on this together, and I know my body better than anyone else.

This is who to contact:
Joan Skyler
Santa Cruz County Public Health

Thank you so much for considering this plan.
Sincerely,

Nicolas

Nick was in the hospital for five days before he was able to negotiate his release. His liver function was twenty times normal. The doctors ran every test imaginable and could not find the reason for this. He itched all over, he was nauseous and very weak. His weight dropped to 128 and as of December 3, his CD4 count was 1.

In spite of his frail health and miserable condition, he decided to go to Wisconsin with Kim and her family for Christmas. Three days before he was to leave, his mother went to his house and found him depressed and lying in bed. He was angry with the medical system that not only wouldn't find the cure, but couldn't even figure out what was wrong with him, let alone treat it.

Luellen suggested that he try peptide T again. Nick was against it, just another one of Mom's goofy ideas. She reminded him that when he took it the year before, in ten days his CD4 count went from 17 to 46. This, she told him, could be due to only one of three reasons: (1) It was a fluke and there was nothing they could do to recreate a fluke; (2) it was the result of the combination of the DDC which he was also taking at the time and the peptide T; or (3) it was the peptide T only.

This argument seemed to get through, but he was still reluctant. His mother climbed on to the bed with him and took his hand in hers and gently and lovingly said, "Remember when I first found out about the at-risk behaviors you where indulging in. I didn't say, 'How could you?' I didn't say, 'That's immoral.' I didn't say, 'Live your life my way.' I said, 'Jon, that's about the best way I can think of for you to get AIDS.' And you laughed at me and said I was just a mother and what did I know. If you had listened to me then, you might not be sick today. Maybe you should listen to me, now."

He nodded and got up. They went to the buyers club in San Francisco and got a fifteen-day supply of peptide T.

The trip to Wisconsin was a long and arduous one for Nick. He required a wheelchair at the airport. Kim's mother, Kenny, called ahead to make sure that wheelchairs were waiting at Denver, where they had to change planes, and in Milwaukee. On the plane Nick felt dreadful and vomited into the airsick bag. He felt bad that Kim and her mother agonized for him, seeing how miserable he was and knowing how uncomfortable and embarrassing it is to be sick in a public place. But Nick took it in stride. He was quite practiced at being ill and could even use the airsick bag without much assault to his dignity.

Wisconsin was a winter wonderland. It had snowed, on cue, just for Nick's arrival. Nicolas hadn't much favored the holidays because the California version didn't fit his images. But the snow-blessed country farmhouse of Kim's grandparents, situated on a frozen lake and warmed by a blaze in the fireplace, and the smells of cookies baking in the kitchen was exactly what Nick thought Christmas should be.

Nick had feared that a trip to America's heartland might put him in the midst of narrow-minded folks who couldn't or wouldn't be able to handle the fact that he had AIDS. His fears were unjustified. Kim's grandparents were loving, Christian people who judged no one. They accepted Nick as he was.

On the trip home, he felt energized enough to refuse the wheelchairs and had no need for the airsick bag. Kim and Kenny were amazed at how well he looked. It was, he said later, the best Christmas of his life, and he was very happy to get home.

Nick's Journal
January 1993

Lately it's been very hard to motivate myself to write—so I'll just gibber here for awhile. I once said that my life has been a series of visions. It seems even more so now. I feel very confused about where I am exactly with my illness. I wish that I could stick a quarter into the slot for a dispensation of my current diagnosis. I just want to know how sick I am. At this moment, aside from having stayed up all night, and being constantly in fear of throwing up whatever precious food I've had — I feel pretty good. But then there's the itching. That's why I've been up all night; itching.

The doctors tell me that my gall bladder is not only enlarged and constricted but filled with "sludge" as well.

It seems that excess bile is being produced in the liver and then through the gall bladder which is where I think most of the trouble is. There's so much bile that it constricts and enlarges and then seeps out to the underside of my skin. Thus, the itching.

Oh god, it's absolutely horrible, this constant itching, everywhere. I've got scabs and cuts, bruises, and scars all over my body from scratching, and there doesn't seem like there's anything I can do. The removal of the gall bladder has been brought up but no one is sure that this would work, but I need to do something . . . anything.

I've finally started to think about writing my autobiography. I've even churned out a couple of wretched paragraphs. I think that the format will be very short essays with free form, quick narrative. The way I used to write when people said I was a talented writer, not just another person with AIDS. Being sick all the time can be a real drag.

After Nick had been on peptide T for two weeks, he reported that his neuropathy seemed better and that he was able to go two days without any pain medication. It seemed that his appetite was improving, too, and he had more strength than he did before. Still nauseous, but less so than before, he had fewer fevers and night sweats. Unfortunately, the jaundice and the itching were worse than ever. Nearly his entire body was covered with sores from the scratching.

The itching drove Nick crazy. Desperate, he called his mother. "Mom, I can't stand this itching any more," he screamed. "I've made up my mind. If it doesn't stop in one week, I'm going to kill myself."

"Nick, calm down," Luellen urged. "Suicide is too drastic a measure."

"You don't understand! If this is how I have to live, then I don't want to live."

"I know, I know," she said. "There is nothing more maddening than itching all the time, but killing yourself is not the answer."

"It'll make the itching stop!"

"Do you want me to come and get you?" she said.

"No, I want the itching to stop."

"I know. Listen, promise me that you will not do anything foolish tonight, and I'll be over the first thing in the morning and we will do something. Okay?"

"Okay."

"Do you promise?"

"I promise I will not kill myself tonight."

When his mother picked him up the next day, he was somewhat quieter, but still agitated. And still itching.

Dr. Polanski prescribed questran to alleviate the itching. He wrote on the prescription, "As needed for itching." According to the pharmacist, MediCal wouldn't cover questran for itching, only for cholesterol reduction. Kim had to pay for the prescription, as Nick was out of funds that day — ninety-seven dollars!

On the day Arthur Ashe died of pneumocystic pneumonia, Nick was in the hospital with pneumocystic pneumonia. The Thursday before, his mother had taken Nick up to San Mateo County General because something was wrong with his lungs. He was weak and his finger nails were white, a sign that the level of oxygen in his blood was too low. The first thing Nick and his mom saw when they arrived in the emergency room was a sign that said: "The wait to see a doctor is 5 hours."

They explained to the triage nurse that Nick had AIDS, that his oxygen level was low, and he couldn't wait five hours.

Then they waited. They waited for an hour. His mom got up to remind the nurse that they were still there. Nick was angered by his mother's impatience, and he got up to stop her. He must have gotten up too fast, because he collapsed in her arms. They were then put in a treatment room right away.

One of the nurses came in and started to take Nick's vital signs. "Hey," he said to her, "you better put some gloves on."

"I'm only taking your pressure and listening to your lungs," said the nurse.

"Can't you see my body is covered with open sores?" said Nick, quite matter-of-factly. "I'm sorry, but I can't let you touch me without gloves. It's for your own protection."

Suddenly, the nurse realized the situation. No one had told her she was working with an AIDS patient.

Another nurse came in, and Nick asked her if he could have a rolled bandage and some sodium chloride that he saw in an open storage locker.

"Sure," she said. "Why?"

"I want to wrap up my legs because they're bleeding."

On the sheet beneath him were several drops of blood. Each drop was encircled by a golden halo of bile. Nick would scratch a particularly bothersome area, and first, yellow powder would just seem to flake out of his skin. Then, as the epidermis layers started to break down, yellow liquid would ooze out and, finally, as the skin was completely torn, blood flowed. The drops of blood and bile would fall to the sheet and separate, with the blood in the middle, framed by the bile.

The nurse helped him wrap his legs, and it seemed that the sodium chloride did offer relief from the itching.

Nick had a chest X ray, some blood work, and a treatment to clear his breathing passages. They gave him azithromycin and told him see his doctor the next morning.

On Friday, Bill took him to the clinic in San Mateo. Dr. Polanski admitted Nick to the hospital. He had pneumonia. His mother was summoned. But by the time she arrived, Nick was very feisty and full of fight.

February 6, 1993

Dear Bubbie and Poppop,

Hello! I wish that circumstances were better, but as luck would have it, I'm writing to you from a hospital bed. I truly wish that I could tell you that everything is fine, but I'd be a liar if I did.

Otherwise, my spirits are high. My feeling is that I need to be an optimist, but that it is both practical and important for me to be a realist as well.

Now, first of all, I can't seem to thank you enough for helping to pay for my alternative treatment, but I'll say it anyway; thank you so very much.

I spoke to Ellen, yesterday. We had a great talk. It seems that she wants to help out as much as she can, but I'm sure you already know that.

This is turning out to be one of the longest hospital stays I've had and I'm very sick right now.

Yet, hopes are high and I'm on my way.

Thank you.

Love,
Jonathan

The video documentary, *Not Me,* Innocence in the Time of AIDS, which Nick had been in, was scheduled to be shown in central California the third week of February. The cast and production crew planned to have a private screening of the documentary, first. As Nick was in the hospital, they gathered in his room to watch it with him. A TV news crew came and interviewed Nick and the other young people in the video. They ran the interview that night on the news. Nick rather enjoyed his celebrity status.

Nick was lying in his hospital bed with his father and the rest of the cast in his room. They were wearing masks, because there was a chance that Nick had tuberculosis, too. The television reporter asked Nick about his condition. He looked up into the camera and said, "I'm not on death's door. I'm going to get through this pneumonia and I'll be fine in two or three months."

Nick was quite pleased with the documentary. In it, he told his story in his own words.

It's hard for me to tell my story, sometimes, because I'm not sure what's the most important part ...

I have a girlfriend that I live with, and I've been dating her for about two and a half years. She gets tested regularly. She stays negative. She loves me. We were dating before I found out about my status and we dated afterward.

Someone said to me once, "If my girlfriend tested positive, I'd dump her." What if you love that person? What if you find out you are in love with someone who has HIV? Does that make a difference? You just watch what you are doing, you take care of yourself and you don't be stupid.

She stayed with me. She slept on the hospital floor when I had pneumonia. She's worked with me. She's not stupid, she doesn't want to catch AIDS. She doesn't want to catch HIV. But she maintains a little decency in her life. We have sex and we are safe and she gets tested regularly.

When I was fifteen years old, I got really drunk one night at a party and lost my virginity and I went crazy afterward. It was like a whole new universe opened for me and so I milked it for all it was worth.

It was funny because at that time, in the mid-'80s, people were educated about AIDS to the extent of: wear a condom. It just didn't dawn on me that it was going to be a problem.

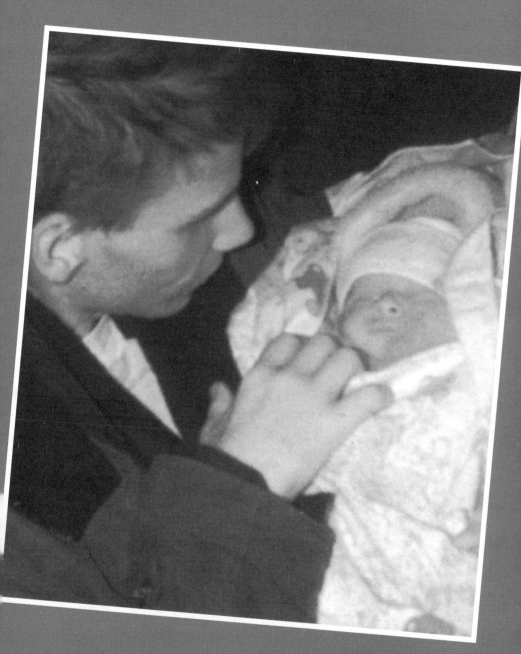

Nicolas about five months before he died, with his
newborn nephew, Anthony. "I wish I could see him
grow up," Nick commented.

By the time I was eighteen, I'd really gotten out there. I was still having sex. I thought about AIDS to the extent of it wasn't something I was ignoring, but it still just didn't dawn on me that it could be me. I hadn't faced that.

Well, life goes on and as I grew older, I felt my life was beginning slowly to take a little bit of form and I decided to go to college. I met a girl and I fell in love and we moved in together and we were beginning to start a wonderful relationship when I started getting sick.

She used to say that she just loved to fall asleep in my arms because I was so warm. I was having fevers of 103 and 104 every night. We didn't even think about it; we knew nothing about medicine or anything. Pretty soon, she starts saying, "You should see a doctor."

Well, that wasn't going to work for me. I didn't have any insurance. I didn't have any money. I didn't think that poor people could get health care. They still pretty much can't, but I made an appointment at the county hospital and they said they'd see me in three weeks.

But I started getting sicker and sicker and I got sicker and pretty soon, I couldn't stand up anymore. My girlfriend put me on her back pretty much and dragged me into the emergency room.

They sat me down and asked me a long list of questions and they told me to open my mouth. I had this stuff in my mouth, this thrush, a fungal infection. They asked me, "Are you HIV-positive?"

And I said, "I couldn't be. I don't know. Am I? You tell me."

[I ended up] in a hospital bed, tubes sticking in my arms, tubes in my nose, people drawing blood every hour. A woman comes in the next day and says, "You have AIDS."

And I said, "How long do I have to live? What happened to this HIV-positive period I was told about where you're okay for years? Why can't I be okay for years? Why is this starting now? Everybody else gets their little five-year period. What about mine?"

They said, "We're sorry, you've had yours."

And I lived in the hospital for two weeks. My family came, my girlfriend came, her family came, my friends came — and they all stood around me. Nobody knew what to do.

But time progressed and I took the medication they told me to take. And eventually I got past that pneumonia that I had and then I had to deal with it emotionally.

I can't really put it into words well. It was a transition like you wouldn't believe and eventually after about six months I got to the point where I could smile. I started going out. I started talking to people.

I still have my bad days, and fortunately I have someone to lean on on those bad days. Sometimes she wants to slap me in the face. I am not exactly the best person to deal with when I'm sick. I have a lot of symptoms. I get sick a lot and I deal with it and when I can't deal with it, I cry.

I have someone who's there for me and I'm getting through this.

With newer treatments, AIDS patients are living longer and longer. But with no cure on the immediate horizon, AIDS remains, ultimately, fatal. The easiest way to avoid infection is to avoid at-risk behaviors such as sex and IV drug use. If you do have sex, use a condom every time so that body fluids are not exchanged. If you use IV drugs, don't share needles —and try to enter a program that will help you become and stay clean. ("Teens Talk . . . About AIDS" (San Francisco: Impact AIDS, Inc., 1993) and "Abstinence & HIV (Santa Cruz, Calif.: ETR Associates, 1992.)

CHAPTER TWELVE

Making
Compromises

Nick phoned his mother to discuss another move. "You remember we talked about me coming to stay with you guys for the summer while Kim does her internship in the city?" he said.

"Yes, I remember."

"Well, Kim and I have been talking, and we decided it would be a good idea for me to stay with you." Nick hated the idea of going home to his parents, but there was no alternative.

"Wonderful," said Luellen. "We'd love to have you. When do you want to come?" The delight in his mother's voice was no comfort to Nick. He was afraid once he was in her house, he'd be in her grip, too.

"Right now. Would it be too much of a problem for you to pick me up tonight and then come back on the weekend and get the rest of my stuff?"

"No it wouldn't be too much trouble," she said. Nick usually did things on the spur of the moment. "I'll be there in forty-five minutes."

She picked him up that night and a few days later, Nick,

his mom, Liz's boyfriend Marty, and Liz went to Santa Cruz, loaded his stuff into Marty's truck, and brought all of it home.

A short time later, Bill went to the buyers' club in San Francisco to get more peptide T for Nick, but they were all out. It could be up to four weeks until they got more. Nick only had a three- or four-day supply left. But Nick would not let himself worry about this fact, even though his mother was convinced that peptide T was the only thing keeping him alive.

The next week, his mom called the buyers' club again. Still no peptide T. They referred her to the Atlanta Buyers' Club, but Atlanta had only twenty-four vials left, which they were saving for their regulars. They suggested calling New York; New York didn't have any, either. The FDA was evidently behind this sudden shortage.

Bill called the manufacturer of peptide T. They told him that with a letter from Nick's doctor, they could possibly distribute the medication to Nick with FDA approval. Dr. Polanski was in Berlin at the AIDS Conference and then he would be taking the rest of the month off.

Nick watched the news about what was going on at the AIDS Conference. There was lots of talk, but no great advances were reported. He leaned forward, intent on every word that emanated from the television. When the report was over he sat back, deflated. "Okay, they can't find a cure. But can't they just keep us alive until they do find one?" he asked.

During the first three weeks Nick was with his parents, his condition improved slightly. But since he'd run out of the peptide T, he wasn't improving as much as before. In June, his anemia worsened and the night before his sister's baby was to be baptized, he went into the hospital to get a blood transfusion. Bill got up at 6 A.M. to rush up to the hospital in San Mateo, taking Nick's clothes with him, to get Nick and bring him back in time for the baptism. Nick was so proud to be Anthony's godfather. He needed the wheelchair that day. Some days he needed the wheelchair and some days he didn't.

Nick was all dressed up in a suit and tie. Kim had purchased the suit for him while he was still living in Santa Cruz. But he didn't have a shirt and a tie, so the week before the baptism his mom took him to the outlets for a little shopping excursion.

First, they went to the shirt store and picked out a white shirt. The problem was finding one in Nick's size. The salesperson measured Nick's neck, and it was not quite 13 inches. Two years before, he had worn a 15 $\frac{1}{2}$.

"I think you might have better luck finding a shirt to fit in a children's store," the salesgirl said. This simple comment forced a look of chagrin on Nick's face.

"Just bring us the smallest one you have," his mother said.

Then they drove two blocks to Brooks Brothers to find a tie. Luellen heaved the wheelchair out of the trunk, wheeled it around, and helped Nick get into it. His feet were very swollen and painful to the touch. Try as she might, she always seemed to bump his feet and hurt him. Nick was patient with her, but he wished his mother wasn't such a klutz.

Nick was more of a Goodwill kind of dresser than a Brooks Brothers type, but for this special occasion he decided to go to Brooks Brothers for a tie. Nick and his mom went from display table to display table and must have touched every tie in the store. This one was too bright, that one too staid. Finally, he picked out a rather conservative blue paisley tie.

"Nick," his mother said, "do you want to wear a blue tie with a black suit?"

He became quite peeved with her, putting the tie back on the table and snapping, "Okay, you pick out whatever tie you want."

"Well, I just meant —

"No, you get the tie that makes you happy."

"Come on, Nick," she said. "I was just making a suggestion." They were receiving looks of disdain from everyone in the store. She was, after all, arguing with an invalid in a wheelchair.

"You're right. This tie is fine."

When they got to the cash register, Nick was too weak to write his own check, so Luellen wrote it and he signed it. His hands were shaking so badly that his name was completely illegible. Nick was relieved that the salesperson didn't say anything except, "Thank you very much, sir. Please come again."

Nick and his mom had settled into a workable, if not pleasant, routine. Each morning, she would come into his room shortly after he awoke and empty his urinal, fill his water pitcher, get his breakfast, and lay out his vitamins and medications for him. They'd visit a while and then she went off to work. She would return at noon and get his lunch, and then again when her workday ended at five. By that time, Nick was usually feeling well enough to get up, so Mom would help him get dressed, and he'd move into the living room for the evening. After dinner he would chat with the family or watch TV. Then his mom would get him cleaned up and ready for bed. She would massage his feet, rub his back, and read to him. Nick could see that she luxuriated in the opportunity to "mother" him. He was at once grateful for her attention and peeved that it was necessary.

In the middle of June, Bill's sister Ellen, her husband, and their two children came to visit. Nick was very happy to see his aunt and uncle and his cousins, Sam, fifteen, and Margot, thirteen, but his behavior was suddenly quite disruptive.

He was taking a lot of dilaudid for the pain in his feet, and the drug had a very adverse affect on his demeanor. He was acting like a spoiled brat. He and Elizabeth got into an argument in front of their guests, and then they wrote "I'm sorry" notes and passed them to each other while the family was sitting and chatting in the living room.

Nick's cousin Sam, who hadn't seen Nick in a year and a half was stunned by the change in Nick's appearance and kept saying, "What happened to him?"

One day they all piled into two cars and drove down to

Carmel to do the tourist thing. They went to lunch and cruised the tourist shops. Although they had brought the wheelchair with them, Nick wanted to walk. He didn't get very far, though, before he fell. Marty was right behind him and caught him. He helped put Nick in the wheelchair, but the incident embarrassed Nick.

Overall, though, the day was enjoyable, but tiring. Nick slept part of the way home. When the rest of the family went to Santa Cruz to the boardwalk the next day, Nick and his mom stayed home.

The following week, his mother took Nick to the clinic for a checkup. The news was not good. The medical community had given up on Nick. Nick understood what was beginning to happen, but his mother needed to be told. "He's dying," his doctor said. "Just take him home and make him as comfortable as you can."

He had a GI (gastrointestinal) bleed, which could clear up or get worse. If it worsened, it would kill Nick in a matter of hours. If it didn't, it would kill him in four or five days. If the GI bleed didn't kill him in a few days, then his anemia would kill him in two or three weeks. If the doctors kept giving him transfusions so he wouldn't die of anemia, then he would die of liver failure in a couple of months.

All of his liver functions were high, except albumin, which was dangerously low. The low albumin was the reason for his edema (swelling caused by water retention). Albumin is the substance that allows the body's tissues to distribute and hold water appropriately. That was why he was swollen with water retention and, at the same time, why his skin was so dry that it was flaky.

Nick's liver was about twice its normal size. It was tender to the touch and he had a lot of abdominal pain. He also had edema in his feet, which moved to his midsection only when his feet were elevated, which is what the doctors told him to do.

When they got home, much to Nick's chagrin, his mother

began to research ways to counter the dire predictions. She told Nick she had found that when the liver is deprived of the digestive enzymes it needs to properly digest protein, it becomes enlarged, tender to the touch, and causes abdominal pain. If it doesn't get enough properly digested protein, it can't produce albumin, which in turn causes edema. For two years, Nick had been taking medications that destroy digestive enzymes.

She started giving him capsules of digestive enzymes after each meal. She also gave him predigested amino acids, because he was having trouble eating enough protein. Nick reluctantly went along with her "prescriptions." He knew it would make her feel better if he took these remedies, but he was skeptical about whether they would help him.

The doctor prescribed Zantac for the GI bleed, but he said he had no idea if it would help with the bleeding or not. Fortunately, it did.

Dr. Polanski was still in Europe and his replacement was a well-intentioned man whom Nick neither liked nor trusted. The replacement doctor sent the VNA Hospice nurse to explain to Nick and his parents how dying at home works. They had no idea the doctor had planned to do this and were completely unprepared for it. Nick was shocked and explained to the nurse that his usual doctor was still in Berlin at the AIDS Conference and that he was dealing with a substitute. "This doctor doesn't know how resilient I am," Nick said. He was still fighting to stay alive. He refused hospice care.

The VNA nurse called the next day to report that when she told the replacement doctor Nick had declined the services of hospice, the doctor told them Nick was incompetent to make that kind of decision and that his parents should decide for him. When Nick's mom told him about the phone call from VNA, he was angered and scared. He did not want to be deemed incompetent. He did not want to lose what little control he had left over his life. Finding that his mother was on his side was a big relief.

"Don't worry," she told him. "We'll fight this. We won't let anybody make these decisions but you. The head of the VNA is coming to assess you herself. All you have to do is show her how competent you are."

"Okay," said Nick. He was determined to win this battle.

The head nurse came to the house and interviewed Nick. He easily convinced her of his ability to make his own decisions, and that was that.

A few days later, Nick's grandfather called. Nick could overhear his mother talking to him in the next room. "No, I am not preparing myself for his death," she said, her voice tense and raised. "I am fighting to keep him alive." She paused to listen and then said, "I will have plenty of time to mourn when he's gone. Right now he is alive." Then her voice lowered and Nick could not hear the rest of her side of the conversation.

Suddenly, he was filled with compassion for his mother. She came into his room a few minutes later, with a smile on her face as if nothing had happened.

"Are you all right?" Nick asked her gently.

"Yes, I'm fine," she said.

AIDS has changed the face of dying. Never before, at least not during peacetime, have so many young people been required to prepare for their own deaths. AIDS is the leading cause of death among those twenty-five to forty-four years old. As of November 1995, more than 501,000 cases of AIDS had been reported in the United States. The World Health Organization estimated that this number was four and a half million on a worldwide basis. In the United States, more than 311,000 deaths have resulted from the diseases that attack those with compromised immune systems, and that figure is ten times greater globally. ("The Names Project," June 1996.)

CHAPTER THIRTEEN

The Final Acceptance

Dr. Polanski returned from Europe, and on July 6 Nick went to see him. They chatted for a while. Then the doctor ordered some blood work and signed a letter to the FDA asking for peptide T for Nick. After Nick and his mom left the office, they went to Peninsula Labs, the manufacturer of peptide T and hand-delivered the letter. The reason Nick's fevers, night sweats, and anemia were worse was because he was out of peptide T.

After they ran that errand, they went to Tower Records because Nick wanted to get the new U2 compact disc. This was the only part of the outing that Nick enjoyed.

Two days later, Nick was in Sequoia Hospital, receiving his third blood transfusion in a month. The day before, his mom had called Dr. Polanski's office for his blood-test results. His hemoglobin was 5.7, less than half of normal. Nick immediately understood the full impact of the situation. Sitting up in the hospital bed rented for him, he looked around the room, almost as though he were looking for something. A sense of fear flashed through his soul, and then he forced himself to relax. Soon he actually felt serene. After a minute or two, he said to his mother, "I need to get my documents in order and I need to plan my funeral."

She nodded.

"I want to be cremated," he said.

"Okay," she said.

"It's very important to me that I'm kept in the right place," he said. "I want to be scattered at Big Sur, but I think that would cost too much."

"Don't worry about that. If you want to be scattered at Big Sur, that's what we'll do. We will do whatever you want."

"Big Sur is my first choice. But if you can't scatter me there, maybe you could put me in the Buddhist Temple in Santa Cruz. I liked that place," he said.

"Don't worry. We'll scatter your ashes at Big Sur."

"I don't want to be sitting on somebody's mantle, you know."

"Jonathan, you will not be in the urn, just your ashes. You," she said, "are going back to your creator."

"Yes, I know that," he said.

They were quiet for a while. Then he asked, "How low does a person's hemoglobin have to be before that person dies?"

"Zero," Luellen answered. He knew she was making up an answer, but he accepted it.

Then he asked, "How does someone die when they have no hemoglobin?"

"Well, first you'd get light headed and silly, maybe dizzy, and then you'd go into a coma and die. It would really be painless and a lot easier than other ways. Why do you want to know?"

"Oh, no reason," he said.

"Are you giving up?" Luellen asked.

"No," he said, "I'm not giving up, but I am accepting the situation the way it is."

Thoughts filled his mind. Finally, he said, "I've had a good life and I'm ready when it's time."

Shortly after that, they left for the hospital. On the way, Luellen told him his courage and tenacity were inspiring to her. That pleased him. "I take a lot of pride in my courage and tenacity," he said.

Kim came to visit him in the hospital. The sight of her always made him happy. When Kim left, Luellen followed her into the hall. Nick knew his mother was going to tell her how bad the situation was.

#

Nick was in an AIDS ward. His roommate was a gay man in his thirties named Evan. He had had Kaposi's Sarcoma. During the day, Evan's parents were there with him, but in the afternoon his lover called to say he would be over later. Evan's parents left then so that they wouldn't have to see Greg, the lover. How cordial and how sad it all was to Nick that the people who loved Evan couldn't support each other.

That night, Greg came and helped Evan on to the commode. Then he cleaned him up. He fed Evan his dinner, washed his face and hands, brushed his hair and teeth, and got him comfortable. Then Greg began to read to Evan from one of those silly romance novels. He would stop every line or two and make a comment or a joke. Nick could hear the two of them through the curtain between their beds. Evan and Greg would giggle at the funny passages and then Greg would go back to reading.

"Listen," Nick said softly to his mother. "Isn't that beautiful. I'm so moved by how much they love each other. That's real love." Nick had tears in his eyes. When the transfusion was over, he and his mother went home to continue the search for peptide T.

July 9, 1993
FAX to: Randy Wycoff, M.D.
Office of AIDS Coordination
U. S. Food and Drug Administration
Dear Dr. Wycoff,

As the attached letter indicates, my son is in need of peptide T to alleviate the pain and symptoms of his HIV infection. Please approve his doctor's request for IND use of this medication as soon as possible, and FAX your approval to Donald Polanski.

Also, I implore you to do what you can to expedite the approval of this drug as soon as possible. I know it is not a cure, but it does greatly improve quality of life and it is not known to be toxic.

Thank you for your time and attention to this matter.

Sincerely,

Luellen Reese
Mother of Nicolas Trevor

Attached letter:

Randy Wycoff, MD
Office of AIDS Coordination
U. S. Food and Drug Administration
5600 Fishers Lane
Rockville, MD 20857

Dear Dr. Wycoff,

I am requesting an exemption for my patient, Nicolas Trevor, so that he may be given peptide T.

Mr. Trevor has been using this medication for about six months and in that time has experienced complete *cessation of his peripheral neuropathy pain. Prior to taking the peptide T, Mr. Trevor had frequent nausea and almost complete loss of appetite. He also suffered from daily fevers and night sweats. With the use of peptide T, his nausea disappeared, his appetite returned, allowing him to gain over 20 pounds in three months and the severity and frequency of his fevers and night sweats were reduced significantly.*

Since Mr. Trevor has been unable to obtain peptide T for three weeks, his neuropathy pain has returned as have the daily fevers and night sweats. Mr. Trevor is also experiencing appetite difficulties.

Please approve my request at your earliest convenience so that Mr. Trevor may again experience improved quality of life.

Thank you for your attention to this matter.

Sincerely,
Donald Polanski, M.D.

A few days later, Bill and Luellen took a much needed "break" and went to the movies. When they returned home, Nick called them into his room. "I have something very important to tell you," he said. "I want you to know that I have made my peace with my God and I am ready to go."

"I am happy for you," his mother said, but her expression told a different story. "Everyone should be at peace with God, but it doesn't mean that you have to go."

"I know," he said, "but I want you to know that I am ready."

He had completed his journey in life and he was at peace. He was finished. He thought back to a time a week or so after he got out of the hospital after his first hospitalization and he was having a conversation about his relationship with Kim with his mother.

"Do you think I love Kim?" he had asked her.

"Yes, I do," she said.

"How can you tell?"

` "By the way you act when you are with her and how you are always talking about her when you are not with her. Why? Don't you think you are in love with her?"

"I know I am," he said strongly. "But I wanted to know how you can tell when someone is in love. Kim doesn't believe in romantic love. She said her father told her that there is no such thing as love. She says she has feelings for me, but she doesn't know what they are, and I tell her those feelings mean that she is in love with me."

After all they'd been through in three years together, Kim no longer doubted she loved Nick. Nick knew he had taught her to know love, and perhaps he had taught her father to love, too. That was a good accomplishment. And he had accomplished many other things that made him feel good, too. He didn't have to stay and suffer. His had been a good life.

#

Nick called his mother at work on the morning of July 12 to tell her that Dr. Polanski's office called to confirm that he had MAI. They were calling in a prescription, which she was to pick up in a hour or so.

He was upset by the news and didn't want to be alone, so his mother rushed home to be with him. But by the time she got there, he had come to terms with the news and was relaxed. He'd forgotten that his mother was rushing home and was surprised and pleased to see her. "I wasn't expecting you home so soon," he said.

"I figured I'd go get the medication and I decided to stop by on my way."

He nodded and she went to the drugstore. They didn't have enough of the new drug on hand to fill the prescription, so she took what they had.

On Wednesday, July 14, Nick heard his mother calling the FDA, as she had been doing every day for the past five days. He wished that she would give up on her quest for the peptide T. The red tape and put-offs she always got only upset her.

Nick could not get peptide T on a compassionate-use basis because neither his doctor nor the manufacturer were licensed to dispense the medication. The FDA representative said she could put him on the waiting list to participate in an open safety study, but she said that this would take a long time, perhaps months. It infuriated Luellen, but Nick was not surprised or concerned.

By noon, Nick was struggling to breathe. His mother gave him a bronchodilator medication, that gave him some relief. Then she called Dr. Polanski and asked him to order oxygen for Nick. The doctor suggested they go to the nearest emergency room and have the on-call physician call him to coordinate the tests and the ordering of the oxygen.

"We have to go to the emergency room," Luellen explained, and picked up his clothes. "Let's get dressed."

"No," he said. "You can't take me. I would feel better if Dad takes me."

Luellen called Bill, and he was home in an hour. By that time, Nick didn't want to go to the hospital at all. His mother was ready to give in to defeat, but Bill was insistent they go.

While Luellen dressed Nick, Bill brought the wheelchair into his room. Then he wheeled Nick out to the car.

Because you are young, you may think that you are immune to HIV and AIDS. Because you are passionate about life, you may act without thinking things through. But consider this. In 1994 there were between 40,000 and 50,000 new cases of HIV infection reported. Of those, one in two was someone twenty-five years old or under, and one in four was someone twenty or younger. ("The Names Project," June 1996) The statistics in 1996 are equally dismal, with HIV infection growing at a faster rate among teens than among any other group.

CHAPTER FOURTEEN

The Final Battle

Nick and his parents were at the local hospital in five minutes. Luellen wheeled Nick into the emergency room while Bill parked the car. She approached the desk where several hospital employees were doing their paperwork. Without looking up, one of them said, "What can we do for you?"

In a voice that was not too loud, but loud enough for them all to hear, his mom said, "This is my son and he has AIDS. He also has MAI, his lungs are filling up with fluid, and he needs oxygen, NOW."

Hospital personnel moved fast. The nurses had him on a machine to dilate and clear his bronchial passages in minutes. They measured his oxygen saturation level, and it was so low the doctor thought the machine was broken.

As Nick began to breathe more easily, he perked up and felt better. He chatted a little with the nursing staff and the respiratory people while his mother explained the situation to the doctor and told him to call Dr. Polanski.

"I don't know any Dr. Polanski," the doctor said nervously.

"Well, if you'd feel more comfortable," she told him, "you can call our family doctor. He is aware of our situation."

"Who is your family doctor?"

"Dr. Brown."

"Fred Brown?" he said with a hint of relief in his voice. "I know him. I'll call."

He was back in a few minutes with a list of tests Dr. Brown wanted and the news that Dr. Brown ordered Nick be admitted. This small-town hospital did not admit AIDS patients, not because they were prejudiced against them, but because it was easier to ship them up to the county hospital than to equip themselves to treat people with AIDS. For Dr. Brown to admit Nick was a first. Nick was slightly impressed to be the first person with AIDS ever admitted to this hospital, but that didn't change the fact that he didn't want to be there. He was being Nick, although not with his usual vigor.

The emergency room doctor came in and said, "How are you doing?"

"Okay," said Nick. Then he coughed.

"Cover your mouth when you cough in front of me," said the doctor.

Nick replied, "You can't catch what I have by my coughing on you."

"You have TB," said the doctor, indicating that he knew MAI was a form of TB, but also demonstrating that he didn't know anything else about this rare infection.

"Yes, but it is not the kind you can catch, unless your immune system is compromised," Nick advised.

"Well, I might have a cold," said the doctor.

"You're immune system would have to be much more compromised than that," Luellen said.

The doctor glared at the two of them and left the room, but the respiratory therapist wanted to know more and she felt comfortable enough not to wear a mask. Nick was always educating. He told the nurses they didn't have to wear masks, but he wouldn't let them draw blood until they all had on gloves.

The results from the blood count came back, and the news was good. His anemia had completely reversed itself; all of his red blood counts were in the normal range, and higher than they had been after his last transfusion. Well, he wasn't going to die of anemia, at least not in the near future. He was pleased about that, but distracted by trying to breathe through the dilating apparatus.

"You see," his mother said, "the vitamin E, selenium, and ferrous glutamate that I've been giving you is working." He nodded and forced a faint smile.

Next, they were shown his chest X ray. Although Nick's right lung was clear, his left lung was completely full of fluid.

Dr. Brown came at about eight-thirty and went over Nick's meds with Nick and his mom. He decided to continue them as prescribed and to add an I.V. of albumin and an I.V. of a powerful antibiotic from the penicillin family.

Dr. Brown wanted Nick to clarify his orders in case Nick's breathing or heart should stop. Gently, he suggested that Nick's condition was grave. "We can make you very comfortable while you are here, Nick," he said, "but if you get worse, we need to know what kind of measures you want us to take."

Nick was confused at first by the question. "What are you saying?" he asked.

Nick had made it clear from the beginning of his journey with AIDS that he did not want to be kept alive artificially by machines, but wanted to die with dignity. He had completed a durable power of attorney so stating, with instructions itemized, witnessed, and signed.

"Nick," his mother said, "Dr. Brown needs to know that you don't want extraordinary measures taken, just in case."

That he understood. He turned to the doctor and said vehemently, "No coma."

A "no code" sticker was put on his chart, indicating he would not be resuscitated.

The hospital pharmacy did not have most of Nick's medications on hand and the nurses were not familiar with many of them, so Bill went home to retrieve their supply. Luellen taught the nursing staff how to administer them and when.

Then they kissed Nick good night and went home. Nick, exhausted and breathing through a oxygen mask, tried to go to sleep, but he was unsuccessful.

When his mother returned the next morning, he was very frustrated at having been unable to eat his breakfast because his oxygen mask was in the way. His O2 sat (level of oxygen in the blood) was not high enough for Nick to use a nasal mask, so he had a full mask with a big bag on it. All he wanted to know was when could he go home.

"Well," his mother explained, "as soon as you are able to breathe comfortably on a nasal mask, you can go home. The in-home oxygen tanks don't accommodate the big masks."

"How long will that take?" he asked.

"A day or two," she said, kissing him and going to work.

When she came back to see him at lunch, Nick was on the nasal mask, but he said he had been going back and forth between the two. He felt alert. He wanted his appointment book, his wallet, and his New York Times. Luellen went home and got them.

By the time she returned, he was using the larger mask again. Nick said to her, "I didn't get better like you said I would."

"Yes, you did," she said. "The three things that your AIDS doctors said were going to kill you were the internal bleeding, and that stopped; the anemia, and according to yesterday's CBC, that has reversed itself; and the liver function, which has improved so dramatically that you're out of danger with that."

"But look at me," he said.

"Well, your lungs have filled up with fluid, but you can get over this in a few days. I know you can do it," she said. "You've done it before. At some level, you make yourself better. You've even told me that."

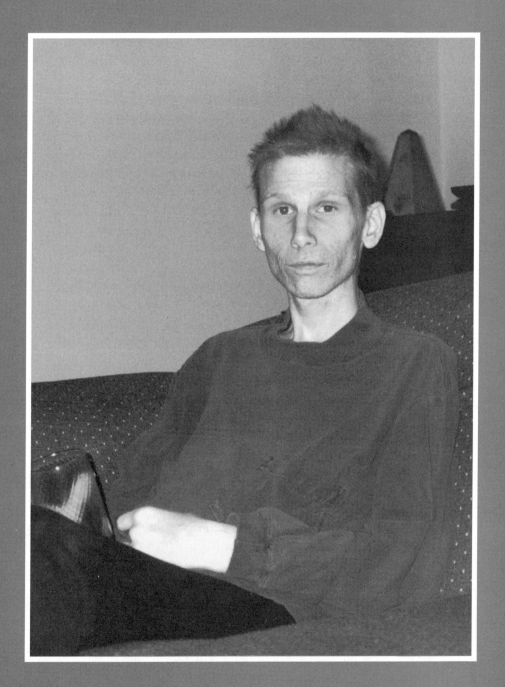

Nicolas about four weeks before he died.

He would have become impatient with his mother, had he not been so tired. He looked at her solemnly. "Mom, when it's time to go, I'm going."

"Yes," she said, "but it's not time yet."

He repeated resolutely, "When it's time to go, I'm going."

That evening, Bill and Luellen went back to see him again and stayed for about two hours. It was hard for Nick to talk because the mask pushed up against his chin. He did say the phone had been ringing that afternoon, but he couldn't reach it to answer it. His mother told him it was Kim calling. He smiled at that. It was enough for him to know she was thinking of him. Luellen said that Kim would be coming on Saturday to visit and he said, "Good."

He was trying to please his mother, but he was finished fighting. Why couldn't she see that? he wondered. He gave her a list of some things that he wanted her to bring him in the morning and then at eight-thirty, his parents got ready to leave.

Nick knew he would never see his parents again. He also knew he could not die with them in the room. It was hard for him to say good-bye to them for the last time, but he knew it would be harder if they knew. He looked at his dad. "Good night," he said. "I love you."

His father bent down and kissed him. "I love you, too, Nick."

Then Nick turned to his mother. He was filled with a warm, radiant love for her. It poured out of his eyes. "Thank you for coming," he said to her.

"Of course," she said, "I'll always come." She brushed his hair with her hand and kissed him on the forehead. "I love you," she said.

"I love you, too, Mom."

Nick waited several minutes, long enough for his parents to be safely out of the building, then he buzzed the nurse and calmly said, "I'm dying." The respiratory therapist came and tried to clear his bronchial passages, but couldn't. Two nurses stayed with him, holding his hands and talking to him. He tensed up a little, then he completely relaxed. The nurses kept talking and comforting him. Nick stopped listening to them, and then he was gone.

Nicolas Jonathan Trevor died at 9:15 on July 15, 1993, of respiratory failure. He died as beautifully and courageously as he had lived.

Epílogue

We received the call from the hospital and rushed back. We parked, ran into the hospital, and up one hall and down the next. The door to Nick's room was closed. I saw the doctor coming toward me. He shook his head. "He's gone," he said.

I stopped for a split second and then said, "Is he in there?" I pointed to his room. The doctor nodded and so I went in.

I felt horror as I saw his lifeless body lying in the bed. It was limp and seemed so small. It was yellow and thin and sunken. The skin had lost its texture. His eyes were caved into his head, and they stared off into nowhere. His mouth gaped open, helplessly.

I wanted to hold him because I knew I would miss holding him. I leaned down, picked him up, and held him tightly. It felt like Jonathan and it smelled like Jonathan, but I knew, I could sense that it wasn't Jonathan I was holding. Jon was not there. He was gone. I sat down next to the bed and put my hand on his arm. I talked to him, and I talked to God for a while. I can't remember what I said, but it was good-bye.

We were blessed that Jonathan did not suffer long or nearly as badly as so many people who died of AIDS. He had made his peace with his God, he knew he was dying, and, as he told Bill and me the Saturday before he died, he was happy and ready to go. He knew he was loved, and he was courageous and tenacious until the end.

Jon's funeral was news as a result of his participation in the documentary, Not Me. We played some of Jonathan's favorite music as the people were arriving. My dad, a Catholic priest, opened the service with a greeting and a call to celebrate Jonathan's life and memory. Then Kim read a poem that Jon had written shortly after they had met. It ended with a line about driving off together in a car, and Kim looked up and said, "and now he's driving away."

Jon's cousin, Christopher, read the speech that Jon had made at the end of the Not Me documentary. We had copies of the speech printed, and Jon's cousins, Lauren and Richard, passed them out to the people before the services began, along with red AIDS ribbons. Elizabeth read a passage from one of Jon's Buddhist books. The passage had been highlighted, so we felt that it was important to him.

Then, Bill read the Mourner's Kadish, first in Hebrew and then in English. He also read a prayer for a dead child and led the gathering in the Serenity Prayer. It's a simple prayer: "God, grant me the serenity to accept the things I cannot change, courage to change the things I can, and wisdom to know the difference."

Finally, my dad conducted the Catholic vigil for the dead, which included two readings from the New Testament, a eulogy, and a prayer.

People filed by and hugged Bill and me. When the room was finally empty, Bill and I said our last good-bye to Jonathan. It was very hard to let go and to know that we could never look upon his face again.

On Thursday afternoon, we went to the funeral home and picked up Jonathan's ashes and brought them home. Bill had made a shrine to Jonathan in the room that had been his. This is a Buddhist tradition. The shrine included pictures of Jon, some of his favorite things, and some plants and flowers. We put the ashes under the shrine, said a prayer, and lit some of Jon's incense. I think Jon would have liked this very much.

Friday morning, my dad, my sisters, and lots of nieces and nephews all gathered at our house where my dad said Mass for Jon. Then, Kim and her mom and dad and aunt Linda arrived. Kim's mom and my sister, Margaret, were both wearing T-shirts that Jon had designed for *Static* when he and Kim had the magazine. Elizabeth was wearing a promotional T-shirt from the "Not Me" documentary, and Kim's aunt was wearing a T-shirt from last year's AIDS walk, when she walked for Jon.

We loaded into three cars and drove down to Andrew Molera State Park at Big Sur. Jon and Bill had gone camping there last year, and just last spring, Jon had taken Kim and their friend Allyson and her boyfriend camping there, too. It was a favorite place of his.

It was about a mile and a half trek to the beach, and another half mile over sand and rock down the beach to the perfect spot. Bill read the Mourner's Kadish again, and then we opened the box. We each took a handful of ashes and waded into the ocean. I put my hand into the water, opened it, and the water carried the ashes away. We each repeated this process until the ashes were gone.

Nick's Speech

I don't think about dying. I feel at peace with death. You know when the time comes, I'll be ready. I've lived a full, wild, crazy, bizarre life. I didn't miss out on anything. I feel that when my time comes, I'll just relax - and hope that some of the things I've done in my life will have an effect on other people. And I think that's a good thing. You know, it makes me feel strong now, and it makes me want to do everything I can to avoid it as long as possible. Trust me, I'm not saying I want to die. But it makes me strong, and it makes me who I am. And I give that to all of you.

— *from the documentary,* Not Me: Innocence in the Time of AIDS

For Further Information

Books

Landau, Elaine. *We Have AIDS*. New York: Franklin Watts, 1995.

Brackenbush, Marcia, et. al., eds. *The AIDS Challenge: Prevention Education for Young People*. Santa Cruz, Calif.: Network Publications, 1988.

O'Connor, Tom. *Living with AIDS: Reaching Out*. San Francisco: Corwin Publishers, 1986.

Peabody, Barbara. *The Screaming Room*. San Diego, Calif.: Oak Tree Publications, 1986.

Shilts, Randy. *And the Band Played On: Politics, People and the AIDS Epidemic*. New York: Penguin Books, 1987.

Sparks, Beatrice, ed. *It Happened to Nancy*. New York: Avon Books, 1994.

Video

Not Me: *Innocence in the Time of AIDS*. Scott Evers, producer. Santa Barbara, Calif.: Sedwith Pictures; Pyramid Films, distribution.

About the Author

Luellen Reese was born and has lived most of her life in northern California. She has been married for twenty-eight years to Bill Reese, and is the mother of Nicolas and Elizabeth and the grandmother of Anthony. She is active in her local Catholic church, loves sailing, works as an executive assistant for a nonprofit agency, and is an avid reader and an occasional writer. Writing this book was a labor of love.